CW00337551

Key Is
Child Protection for
Health Visitors and Nurses

Other titles from Longman

NSPCC: *Child Sexual Abuse: Listening, Hearing and Validating the Experiences of Children* by Corinne Wattam, John Hughes and Harry Blagg.

NSPCC: *Listening to Children: The Professional Response to Hearing the Abused Child* edited by Anne Bannister, Kevin Barrett, and Eileen Shearer

NSPCC: *From Hearing to Healing: Working with the Aftermath of Child Sexual Abuse* edited by Anne Bannister

Making Sense of the Children Act (2nd edition) by Nick Allen

NSPCC: *Making a Case in Child Protection* by Corinne Wattam

KEY ISSUES IN CHILD PROTECTION FOR HEALTH VISITORS AND NURSES

Edited by
Jane Naish and Christopher Cloke

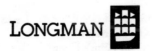

Published by Longman Industry and Public Service Management,
Longman Group UK Ltd, 6th Floor, Westgate House, The High,
Harlow, Essex CM20 1YR, England and Associated Companies
throughout the world.

A catalogue record for this book is available from The British Library

ISBN 0-582-09754-1

Typeset by Anglia Photoset Ltd, Colchester, Essex
Printed and bound in Great Britain by
Biddles Ltd, Guildford and King's Lynn

Contents

*The opinions expressed in this book are those of the individual authors and
do not necessarily constitute the policies or practice of the Health Visitors
Association or the NSPCC.*

List of contributors

Christopher Cloke is Head of Policy Development with the NSPCC, where he has worked for five years. He has been particularly involved in the Society's campaigning activities, which have sought to change public and professional attitudes to children. Prior to joining the NSPCC he worked with a number of voluntary agencies including Age Concern England where he covered health and social services issues.

Jane Naish is currently one of the five Community Health Advisers at the Royal College of Nursing. She has worked as a health visitor in Birmingham and London. She is also a sociologist and has taught at the University of Warwick. She was formerly Professional Officer for the Health Visitors Association, where she had particular responsibility for child protection issues, including the HVA's work on the Children Act and its' implementation.

Tom Narducci is a national training and development officer with the NSPCC. Although born and raised in New York City, his training was in the UK, where he gained a Certificate of Qualification in Social Work. Before entering the field of training, he was a social worker for ten years, first with a local authority and then with the NSPCC.

Jane Parkinson is a health visitor who has previously worked as both a senior nurse manager and a nurse specialist in child protection. She currently works as a psychotherapist in private practice, having trained at the Institute for Self Analysis. Much of her present work is with adults who were abused as children. She lives in Brighton.

Carole Peall is an experienced nurse and in 1988 was appointed child protection co-ordinator for Bolton Health Authority. She previously worked as a health visitor in both Bolton and Wigan.

Robyn Pound, originally from New Zealand, qualified as a health visitor in 1974. She has worked in London, Bristol and Bath, and is an active campaigner for the rights of children in the debate against the physical punishment of children. She published *Help Your Child* *to Sleep* in 1989 and is now reading for a Bachelor's degree in Health Studies.

Jeremy Roche is a lecturer in the Department of Law at the Polytechnic of East London where he has a special interest in child care law. He was closely involved in the production of the Open University training materials on the Children Act and is a member of the management board of the Children's Legal Centre.

Wendy Stainton Rogers is a senior lecturer in the Department of Health and Social Welfare at the Open University, where she had responsibility for the training resource pack on the Children Act commissioned by the Department of Health. She has written and been involved in a number of training resources on child protection issues, including a pack on child sexual abuse for the Royal Society of Health and one on health visiting for the Health Visitors Association.

Peter Tattersall has been a trainer and consultant in the public and voluntary sector for the past seven years. He specialises in courses and workshops on assertion, managing violence, negotiating, teamworking, management, and staff development. He was accredited by the Coverdale Organisation for his work with management teams at the NSPCC. He currently divides his time between freelance work and training and consultancy for Wandsworth Council.

Ben Thomas is Chief Nurse Advisor and Director of Quality at the Royal Bethlem and Maudsley Hospital Special Health Authority. He is also an honorary lecturer at the Institute of Psychiatry, London. One of his special interests is sexuality and gender in relation to nursing, about which he has published a number of articles.

Jim Waters is team manager of the NSPCC Therapeutic Centre for the Child in Warrington, Cheshire. He is a qualified and experienced social worker, and for a number of years was a child protection officer with the NSPCC Child Protection Team in Rochdale. While at Warrington he co-managed a project with specialist health visitors attached to social work child protection teams.

Jane Wynne is a consultant community paediatrician, Leeds Health Authority. She has written and taught extensively on child abuse in general and on sexual abuse in particular. She has been at the forefront in the debate on the diagnosis and assessment of child sexual abuse. She is active in issues relating to children's rights.

Foreword

Child protection in the 1990s is on the threshold of opportunity with the implementation of the Children Act 1989 and the revised government guidelines *Working Together*. The principles underpinning this Act and government guidance *should* have a profound effect on child protection practice and, in turn, on the lives and wellbeing of many children and their families. We use the word 'should' deliberately because at the time of writing it is too soon to say, with any certainty, how the new measures are being put into effect, particularly since there are significant resource and training constraints at present — and probably for the foreseeable future.

Importantly, the Children Act requires a shift in attitudes and culture on the part of professionals and the institutions for which they work. It is all too often these more intangible factors which are most difficult to alter.

There can be no doubt that the key concepts at the heart of the Children Act, which are taken up in *Working Together*, are ideals to strive towards: children as individuals whose rights, needs and welfare are paramount; equality of opportunity and a commitment to anti-discriminatory practice; the importance of preventive services; minimum standards of care, with children, parents and other users having the right to expect services to be of a high quality; participation and partnership, giving children and their families the right to be consulted and involved in major decisions affecting their lives; recognition that parents have responsibilities for their children and the state has responsibilities to children and parents. It is easy to list the principles — putting them into practice is much more demanding.

Ideas and approaches to work become matters of routine in institutions and become difficult to shrug off or adapt. Changes are threatening, because we are not familiar with the desired result, so it is little wonder that we resist and retreat behind 'proven' existing practice which has served us so well over many years. This book explores the dynamics of change in relation to the child protection work of health visitors and nurses.

In responding to the needs of vulnerable children, health visitors and community nurses are not working alone or independently. The importance of professionals from different disciplines co-operating with each other is emphasised in the *Working Together*, guidelines, which state that the duties and functions 'of agencies and associated groups in relation to child protection . . . should be organised in order to contribute to inter-agency co-operation for the protection of children . . . The responsibility for protecting children should not fall entirely to one agency: awareness and appreciation of another agency's role will contribute greatly to collaborative practices.' And yet, social workers generally have the keyworker role with children placed on child protection registers and are the lead child protection profession. They cannot and should not, however, take action independently from other professions. They have experiences to share with health visiting and nursing colleagues.

The nursing professions have a distinct and special contribution to make to tackling child abuse on a number of levels — on a continuum from prevention to involvement in long-term local authority care. The focus of their work will vary, health visitors and school nurses, for example, working particularly on preventive activities and strategies. They see large numbers of children who, for the most part, lead happy, healthy and protected lives. This may mean that they are often well able to identify families under stress and take steps to provide support before situations of abuse develop. They are also well placed to identify children who have been abused, so that the necessary protective action can then be initiated. There is enormous potential.

Paradoxically, however, the health visitor's and school nurse's familiarity with 'normal functioning families', if such families really exist, and their emphasis on preventive work may also place them at a disadvantage. They may be wary of taking steps which will jeopardise the relationships which they have with families — the 'what if I've got it wrong' syndrome. They may lack confidence as to how to respond when they encounter abused and neglected children. Indeed, we may all seek to deny that adults can behave towards children in such ways, either because the boundary of what is acceptable is not clear or because the act is too appalling to contemplate. Moreover, because many of the nursing and medical professionals with whom they work may share a similar perspective, nurses may encounter problems in being heard when they express their concerns. They may need to assert themselves more effectively.

Needless to say, health visitors and nurses are not alone in facing such dilemmas. Teachers, for example, are in a similar position and do not want to undermine the supportive relationship which they have with pupils and parents. The 'confidentiality trap' applies to them too. *Key Issues in Child Protection for Health Visitors and Nurses* explores these challenges of child protection for health visitors and nurses and considers practical solutions.

It also looks at how the community nurses' skills and their approach to families may complement those of other professionals. Consideration is given to how the experiences and techniques of other professionals — particularly social workers — who are more regularly involved in child protection may be modified for nursing practice. This bringing together of such resources helps ensure that the vital link between prevention and protection is forged. We feel that the book will be of great value to both practising and student nurses. The theoretical discussions are counterbalanced with sound practical advice.

It must be remembered, however, that as with all professionals, health visitors, nurses and their colleagues are not practising in a vacuum but in a real world which may contain powerful forces which militate against effective child protection. In this context it must never be left to individual practitioners to protect children — we must all share that responsibility: the professions themselves, managers, employing authorities, professional associations, and everyone as a citizen alike.

Many have long thought that children's health services have been marginalised within the health service for some considerable time. The British Paediatric Association, the Health Visitors Association, the NSPCC and others share concerns that the current reforms to the NHS may lead to a two-tier system, in which there is a danger that children receive a significantly inferior service. The application of economic and market values may limit the accessibility and availability of health care and preventive services. In such a situation there is a real worry that many health professionals will be less able to take protective action in the face of child abuse and neglect. In introducing further reforms, it is vital that these considerations and the principles of the Children Act are not forgotten and that the voice of children is heard. Purchasers must ensure that the contracts with child health service providers always contain provision for child protection. All professionals working with children have a responsibility to ensure that the needs of children and vulnerable families are properly represented.

Key Issues in Child Protection for Health Visitors and Nurses arose in part out of a conference jointly organised by the Health Visitors Association and the NSPCC, held in Manchester at the end of 1991. That conference was a good example of professionals from two different disciplines — nursing and social work — working fruitfully together. This book is another example. While it is not easy to achieve, multidisciplinary collaboration is possible. This book will assist that process in the area of child protection.

Alison Norman, Chair, Health Visitors Association
Christopher Brown, Director, NSPCC
1992

Introduction

The politics of child protection work in nursing practice
Christopher Cloke and Jane Naish

Child abuse has rarely been out of the news recently. In the past decade a year has not passed without a major public inquiry into the death of a child following child abuse or neglect. More often than not, an individual worker — usually a social worker — is the subject of criticism. The practice of other child protection workers, including the medical and nursing professions, has also, at times, been seen to be lacking. The occurrence of these tragedies is probably not so very remarkable to most professionals involved in child protection work, but invariably they are hailed by the media and public opinion as a total surprise — the story line being that professionals are found to be at fault, they have not followed the recognised child protection procedures, and something must be done! An assumption within this is that the procedures can prevent child abuse, are therefore lacking, and need to be recast. But this analysis both ignores the structural influences and the prevailing social mores, and seeks to pathologise those who are accused of abusing children — in short, it is the 'them not us' syndrome. Recent years have seen a plethora of such official reports (Department of Health, 1991a).

One such report, into the death of Doreen Aston, provides a sensitive discussion of the work of health visitors in relation to child protection and analyzes their role more comprehensively than any other child abuse inquiry (Lambeth, Lewisham, and Southwark Area

Review Committee, 1989). The report describes the social context in which Doreen Aston lived her all-too-short life. The Inquiry Panel noted the characteristics of the neighbourhood where Doreen and her family lived: the housing included high-rise council flats, bed and breakfast accommodation for homeless families, and multiple occupied, old and poor quality converted housing. There were inadequate community child care facilities despite the area having a high proportion of single parents, apparently 'immature' parents, and a high proportion of families living in poverty. The violence in families, the panel commented, often resulted in the emotional and physical abuse of children. The panel concluded that in the face of such conditions only crisis intervention could be achieved in health visiting.

And yet, this is the context in which health visiting and community nursing is conducted in many areas. It is a picture which will be familiar to many readers. From this description we can understand some of the pressures experienced by nurses, *and* the families with whom they work, which make child protection work not as straightforward as the official guidelines suggest.

Many of the texts and much of the guidance offered to nurses focus on the procedures and protocols of nursing without giving consideration to the actual dilemmas of child protection work which nurses experience in the real world. Some, but not all, of these issues have been addressed by other professional groups — notably social workers — but very little discussion has taken place within the nursing professions. This is a reflection not just of the fact that insufficient priority is accorded to the role of the nurse in dealing with child abuse within the multidisciplinary network, but also of a failure to analyze the importance of power relations both in general and specifically within nursing.

Key Issues in Child Protection for Health Visitors and Nurses considers some of the issues and dilemmas which nurses and health visitors encounter on an almost daily basis and which, unless addressed, have the potential for making practice not only difficult but also dangerous, in that assumptions based on individualistic or pathological explanations can leave children still at risk of abuse. Factors relating to power, values, beliefs and social norms within society exert a potent influence on nursing practice both generally and specifically in the highly emotive area of child abuse. It is emotive since all workers bring to this area the baggage of their own childhood and subsequent life experiences, their culture, values, sexuality, and the strong influences of other important people in their lives. These factors are all too often taken for granted and ignored. There are very few forums in which such issues can be safely discussed.

This book brings together contributors from a range of backgrounds for the first time to discuss these issues in relation to nursing, and debates both the issues and ways of resolving the conflicts which nurses and health visitors encounter in responding to child abuse.

The importance of child protection work

Although children comprise one of the largest and most vulnerable groups in society, their needs are frequently not recognised or met. And yet, paradoxically, all nurses are charged with the responsibility to ensure that *every* child has the opportunity to reach his or her full potential — physical, emotional and social. Ensuring that children are protected from all forms of abuse is one facet of this work.

A wide range of nurses come into contact with children: health visitors, midwives, school nurses, practice nurses, paediatric nurses, accident and emergency nurses, psychiatric nurses, and nurses for people with learning difficulties. As a matter of course, all these nurses will come across children who may be at risk or who have actually been abused. They not only need to know how to respond — the relevant policies and procedures — but also how to manage the obstacles, both personal and social, which may militate against providing any effective response.

The family of nursing embraces a variety of skills and perspectives. The nursing role in child protection begins with prevention in the widest sense, and includes the promotion of positive parenting and teaching parents and potential parents — including schoolchildren — about normal behaviour and development in children, so that they understand and can anticipate what to expect. This preventive work also includes profiling populations in order to actively seek out families under stress who may need support and ensure that such families actually receive support appropriate to their needs. Such support may be facilitated either by the nurse herself or provided through other means, such as parent and toddler groups, respite care, financial assistance, marriage guidance, counselling and so on.

The nurse also has a role, as part of the preventive remit, in campaigning in the wider society. This will involve pressing for both adequate family and child resources and also changes in societal values, so that the status of parenting is recognised as skilled work and *children are valued as people.* Britain is *not* a child friendly society, as many parents who have taken their children into restaurants or on the London underground will know to their cost, and children are not necessarily valued as equal citizens with full human rights. Nurses *can* campaign for the promotion of children's rights as equal citizens. They can, for example, support EPOCH (the campaign to End

Physical Punishment of Children) — the Health Visitors Association has set an example through its support (Cook et al., 1991).

The role of the nurse also extends to the other end of the child protection continuum in supporting children who are looked after in long-term local authority care placements and providing health care within a child-centred framework which listens to, and values, the opinions of children and young people. Such children often have multiple health needs and problems which must be comprehensively addressed on an on-going basis. All too often their health — and indeed social — needs are overlooked.

From this it can be seen that nurses and health visitors are in contact with a range of families and children in different circumstances. They will certainly encounter children who have been or who are at risk of abuse, and in so doing they will need to take decisions about what action to take. Such cases are never clear cut, and the decisions are not easy, taken as they inevitably are in a wider social context.

The nature of the work will also require many 'gear changes' in nursing practice, from working with a group of mothers in a mother and toddler group to responding to a child who has a bruise which may be non-accidental. Such a variety and range of child protection work is both emotionally taxing and time-consuming, and a number of other competing priorities and demands made by different clients, patients and other professionals also has to be balanced. However, child protection remains an important part of the nursing remit which is not easy to achieve when services are already overstretched. No wonder that nurses and health visitors face dilemmas over how best to respond.

Current definitions of child abuse

The definition and concept of child abuse, as we shall show in detail, is socially constructed, and what is perceived to be abusive behaviour will vary across time and culture. Child sexual abuse, for example, was only included in government guidelines as a category for registration purposes in 1988. And official definitions of abuse may in any case differ from what either the individual professional considers abuse to be and, indeed, from what families or clients understand it to be. Nevertheless, our starting point here will be the recently updated official definitions laid down in the *Working Together* guidelines for professionals to follow in making decisions about the placement of children on child protection registers (Department of Health, 1991c). While child protection workers from all disciplines should, in theory, be working to these definitions, the reality is probably different, since each individual and profession will bring to their work a different set of background expectancies.

Working Together outlines four categories for the purposes of child protection registration:

Neglect: The persistent or severe neglect of a child or the failure to protect a child from exposure to any kind of danger, including cold or starvation, or extreme failure to carry out important aspects of care, resulting in the significant impairment of the child's health or development, including non-organic failure to thrive.

Physical Injury: Actual or likely physical injury to a child, or failure to prevent physical injury (or suffering) to a child including deliberate poisoning, suffocation and Munchausen's syndrome by proxy.

Sexual Abuse: Actual or likely sexual exploitation of a child or adolescent. The child may be dependent and/or developmentally immature.

Emotional Abuse: Actual or likely severe adverse effect on the emotional and behavioural development of a child caused by persistent or severe emotional ill-treatment or rejection. All abuse involves some emotional ill-treatment. This category should be used where it is the main or sole form of abuse.

These definitions seek to group types of abuse. In reality, however, child abuse will rarely be so clear cut and there will be overlap between the different 'types'. The definitions do not really help to identify the narrow line between what is abuse and what is not. That is for the practitioner to judge.

It is important to note, surprisingly, that *Working Together*, which is a national guidance document for professional practice, continues to state that these categories do not coincide precisely with the definition of 'significant harm' as specified in the Children Act 1989 and which will be relevant if court proceedings are to be initiated.

For example, with a case of neglect it will be necessary to consider whether it involves actual or likely 'significant harm' and whether it involves 'ill-treatment' or 'impairment of health or development' (in each case as defined by the Act). The Courts may well provide an interpretation of 'sexual abuse' (which is not defined in the Act) which is different from that used above in particular cases, in which case their definition should be used in relation to those cases. (Department of Health, 1991c.)

Thus, for the purposes of *legal* proceedings, the definition of child

abuse is different in the Children Act from the definition offered by
the government in *Working Together*.

An important point to note is that these definitions almost
certainly bear little resemblance to what the majority of parents will
consider child abuse to be if asked. The concepts also need to be
operationalised by child protection workers who need to be sensitive
to the way in which families present problems — concerns about
sexual abuse, for example, may be expressed in terms which are very
distant from the government definition quoted above.

Important for nurses and health visitors is the fact that the latest
government guidance points to the need for professionals to be
concerned about the *future risk to an unborn child*. This is new. The
guidelines say that 'on occasions there will be sufficient concern about
the future risk to an unborn child to warrant the implementation of
child protection procedures and the calling of a child protection
conference to consider the need for registration and the need for a
child protection plan' (Department of Health, 1991c).

The current edition of *Working Together* also highlights two
emerging concerns about other ways in which child abuse presents —
institutional abuse and *organised abuse*. Both these developments have
attracted interest in the early 1990s following particular cases, notably
the institutional abuse cases in Staffordshire which led to the Pindown
Report (Levy and Kahan, 1991) and the alleged cases of organised
abuse in Nottingham, Rochdale and the Orkneys. Nursing professions need to take account of these developments in their practice.

Working Together states that

> All those involved with the provision of care for children in
> residential settings, including schools, must be alert to the
> possibility of abuse by other children, visitors, and members of
> staff. Policies and managerial procedures must openly recognise
> the possibility of abuse and must prevent creating circumstances
> which could encourage abuse. (Department of Health, 1991c)

There are important considerations for nurses which have hitherto
not been fully acknowledged. The role of the school nurse in relation
to abuse in schools is an obvious example. It might also be argued that
each residential children's home should have a named nurse or health
visitor with responsibility for ensuring that the health care needs of
children are met in that establishment.

In the 1980s professionals working in the area of child abuse faced
considerable resistance to the notion that children could be sexually
abused. In the 1990s the same problem of denial is being experienced
by professionals in relation to organised abuse, particularly ritualistic
abuse. This topic requires further detailed research and it is still too
soon to draw firm conclusions. The *Working Together* definition is

helpful and worth quoting in full:

> organised abuse is a generic term which covers abuse which may involve a number of abusers, a number of abused children and young people and often encompass different forms of abuse. It involves, to a greater or lesser extent, an element of organisation.
> A wide range of abusing activity is covered by this term, from small paedophile or pornographic rings, often but not always organised for profit, with most participants knowing one another, to large networks of individual groups or families which may be spread more widely and in which not all participants will be known to each other. Some organised groups may use bizarre or ritualised behaviour, sometimes associated with particular 'belief' systems. This can be a powerful mechanism to frighten the abused children into not telling of their experiences. (Department of Health, 1991c)

Clearly, there may be some overlap between organised abuse and institutional abuse.

The experience of workers who have handled cases showing characteristics of organised abuse suggest that these cases are qualitatively different from intrafamilial abuse and place additional — and potentially frightening — pressures on the staff involved. There is a strong need for multi-agency collaboration, sometimes involving staff from several neighbouring authorities, since an organised abuse network may cover a large geographical area. The specific role of the nursing professions in response to organised abuse has not hitherto been discussed, but the themes of this book in relation to the dilemmas which nurses face in child protection work will bring into sharp focus the context in which organised abuse may be embedded.

Incidence of child abuse

The actual incidence of child abuse and neglect is not known. We only know with any certainty about *reported* cases of child abuse, and such information is based on either child protection registrations or on surveys which have asked people about their experiences of being abused. Neither approach is free from problems. These result partly from issues of definition — individuals have different perceptions of what constitutes abuse — and also from variations in registration practice across the country. Thus, attitude surveys which have asked people if they have been abused indicate a higher incidence of abuse than the number of child abuse registrations would suggest.

Creighton (1992) notes that 'it should be emphasised that the children placed on registers represent the reported incidence, not the actual incidence of abuse. The registers only record cases identified, and then notified, by the professional network of agencies involved in child protection. Experience suggests that some cases never come to professional attention and others are not notified to the register.'

Significantly, Creighton goes on to suggest:

> The children of the middle classes are less likely to come to the attention of these agencies than the children of the poor and disadvantaged. There is also some evidence that levels of suspicion in professionals are affected by socio economic status. (1992)

Creighton quotes a research study by O'Toole et al. (1983), in which physicians were presented with a vignette concerning a child with a serious injury. When the parents were described as being of a low social status, 70 per cent considered the injury to be child abuse, whereas only 51 per cent judged it to be abuse when the parents were described as of high socio-economic status. Interestingly, nurses and experienced professionals were not affected by the social status of the parents.

Moreover, what we recognise to be child abuse is socially defined. This may account in part, for example, for the current low reporting of emotional abuse. Emotional abuse is found in all social groups but the response to it may vary. Some members of the higher social classes may resolve the problems by sending their children to boarding schools. The under-reporting of both emotional abuse and neglect is a cause for concern.

It is only since 1988, following the Cleveland 'crisis' and the Department of Health issuing the first edition of *Working Together*, that the government has compiled and issued national figures on registrations based on returns made by local authorities. These figures have been updated annually since then. The latest Department of Health figures (1991b) show that there were 43,600 children on child protection registers at 31 March 1990 in England. That is a rate of 4 children per 1000 of the population under eighteen years of age. The proportions of children registered under the different categories were as follows:

Grave Concern	41%
Physical Abuse	21%
Sexual Abuse	15%
Neglect	16%
Emotional Abuse	5%

These figures include 4 per cent of children who were registered in mixed categories — for example, physical and sexual abuse.

It is significant to note that although the largest group of registrations is 'grave concern', the latest government guidelines have abolished this category, and we can only speculate on what will happen to the children who might have otherwise been so registered. It is often cases of this sort about which professionals have most doubt. These are some of the cases which health visitors and nurses will often encounter, and if they are not registered, and therefore not so likely to be allocated to a social worker, a greater responsibility may fall to the health visitors, nurses and other professionals working with children in the community.

The debate about the incidence of child abuse and reports in recent years about 'sharp rises in child protection registrations' has led some people to conclude that child abuse has reached epidemic proportions. This is, of course, a very long way from reality, and the vast majority of children lead happy, safe and protected lives.

The social construction of childhood and child abuse

It may be surprising for some readers to learn that the category of childhood is not in fact static and does not necessarily relate to chronological age. Historical studies have shown that the boundaries of childhood have varied considerably and children have been perceived by society to have reached childhood at different ages in different periods of history. Social perceptions of who is a child, and how such decisions are constructed, change over time and are subject to a range of factors over and above the simple chronology of age in terms of time. For example, Aries (1962) has demonstrated that the idea of childhood did not exist in England in the Middle Ages: children were expected to reach physical autonomy by the ages of five to seven and then to share in the work and play of 'adults'.

Two key factors determining perceptions of childhood are the economy and the culture of the society, and these two influences may intertwine. Economic forces and the need for children or young people to work in order to maintain both the family and the national economy appear to be key influences in determining adult status. Hence shifts in the ages at which children leave school and may be accepted as adults are as much a reflection of the needs of the economy as of the physical and mental maturity of children.

The notion of childhood is, of course, also culturally specific. Different cultures label and determine childhood differently. For some Muslim cultures, for example, childhood is shorter in terms of the time span in comparison with white western cultures.

In the United Kingdom today there are still anomalies within the concepts of childhood and adulthood. Children can leave school at sixteen, but they cannot vote until they are eighteen or be elected members of parliament or local councillors until they are twenty-one, even though they can join the forces and fight and die for their country.

The movement of the boundaries between adulthood and childhood has a direct correlation with definitions of what is, and what is not, child abuse. Young people throughout history have been exploited and injured but this has not always been construed as child abuse or necessarily 'wrong'. Public concern about child cruelty and neglect really surfaced at the end of the nineteenth century as the expression of a number of leading philanthropists and reformers of the day, including Benjamin Waugh who helped found the National Society for the Prevention of Cruelty to Children and who was instrumental in securing the passing of the Cruelty Act in 1889. Social conditions at this time were in a state of great change, with increasing industrialisation and urbanisation which created poor and over-crowded housing conditions. In these circumstances children as a group were more open to scrutiny and began to come under the public gaze. Interestingly, health visiting also has its origins in this period.

Diungwall et al. (1981) have suggested that the concerns about the wellbeing of children in the nineteenth century developed in the context of new ideas emerging about childhood being a state of 'essential innocence corrupted only by social conditions'.

Equally important, however, were deep-seated fears about the instability of the social order and the potential growth in lawlessness and drunkenness. There was also mounting concern about the significant increase in marital disharmony. Against this background, some degree of intervention in family life, in order to protect children from cruelty, came to be seen as justified. However, intervention in child abuse was limited in that any protective measures were dependent upon the prior criminal protection of the parent(s).

But this context is important since present-day child protection work originated from the dominant social attitudes and prevailing conditions of that time. Ferguson (1991) locates many of today's key themes in child protection practice in this period. He writes:

> This [child protection] practice is in reality a century old. In the 1880s, reformers and social workers developed a systematic legal and social child protection practice in response to what they regarded as a major problem of child abuse. By 1908, in the Children Act of that year, a specific child protection practice had been codified and institutionalised into the foundations of the modern welfare state. (1991)

In a fascinating study, Ferguson examines in detail a particular case handled by an NSPCC inspector between 1891 and 1898. With few amendments, the casework of that period could equally well have been practised one hundred years later. At the end of the nineteenth century, NSPCC inspectors related to local NSPCC branches which comprised supporters who had a fundraising role but also, selectively, an input into case management. Ferguson points out that members of the branches included a range of local dignitaries, including the Mayor, the Chief Magistrate and Justices of the Peace. He suggests that 'the character of child protection practice was shaped from the outset through the interplay between the locality, ethnicity, politics, class, and gender' (1991). The same comments can apply equally well in the 1990s.

The next revival of interest in child abuse came in the 1960s on both sides of the Atlantic following the publication of *The Battered Child Syndrome* by American paediatricians Henry Kempe and his colleagues (1962). This influential work based child abuse on a biomedical model of signs and symptoms, and it was argued that a substantial number of cases of abuse were either wrongly or never diagnosed as such, often with serious results. These conclusions were drawn from medical data, and the paediatric profession played a key part in promoting this cause. Kempe contended that child abuse was the result of the defective personalities of the parents, and while some parents were so impaired that they could not be helped, some 80 per cent of abusing parents could be assisted.

In Britain, Kempe's theories gained widespread support from the medical professions, which were eager to maintain their professional influence, and indeed in the mid-60s the British Paediatric Association issued guidance to its members on responding to these cases. Following a visit to the USA by its Director, the NSPCC set up a Battered Child Research Team in 1963 to test out Kempe's ideas.

Dingwall et al. (1981) have suggested the appeal of Kempe's approach was the notion that 'battering begets batterers and, further that violence or neglect suffered in early childhood creates unstable personalities who are a threat to the social order'. Such a view is shared by Parton (1990) who argues that the medical model, based on individual 'disease' and 'treatment', was the prevalent and predominant factor in the 'discovery' of child abuse in the 1960s and 70s. He goes on to suggest that

> debates about the nature of child abuse and what to do about it are at root not technical and professional but political. Essentially they are about how we should bring up children and in particular the most appropriate relationships that can be developed between the state and the family. (1990)

Parton describes child abuse in terms of structural inequality, rather than as a problem of disease in which the focus is on inter-personal relationships and the relevance of social and economic factors denied or minimised.

The death of eight-year-old Maria Colwell, following physical abuse by her stepfather in 1973, was one more turning point (Department of Health and Social Security, 1975). It provoked huge public interest on a hitherto unknown scale. The then Secretary of State for Health, Sir Keith Joseph, commissioned a public inquiry into Maria's death. Just a few days prior to announcing the establishment of the inquiry, Sir Keith had attended the first residential meeting of the 'Tunbridge Wells Study Group' — a group of doctors, lawyers, social workers and other professionals who had come together to consider the battered baby syndrome. At that time Sir Keith was also promoting theories about a 'cycle of deprivation' which, again, centred on the individual and inadequate parenting as being at the root of family poverty. These ideas fitted well into the model of child abuse which focused on the individual pathology.

The 'discovery' of child sexual abuse in the 1980s, culminating with the 'Cleveland Affair' in 1987, is the latest landmark in the history of child abuse. Formal identification of the problem of child sexual abuse also first emerged in the USA. Finkelhor (1979) suggests that, although it was the medical profession which highlighted physical abuse and also sexual abuse in terms of medical signs and symptoms, it was an alliance within the women's movement that focused public attention on child sexual abuse. Parton suggests that the women's movement may also have been influential in the UK. In addition some paediatricians in local areas may also have seen themselves as breaking new ground in the diagnosis of child sexual abuse. Sexual abuse was seen as an act predominantly perpetrated by men — although it should be noted that there is now an emerging debate on the role of women as sexual abusers — and that, in common with other forms of abuse, it constitutes an abuse of power over children by adults.

Paediatricians in Cleveland were seen as diagnosing much higher levels of child sexual abuse than 'really' existed in the community. They were accused of being over-zealous and of over-reliance on medical diagnostic techniques. Two women — the paediatrician, Dr Marietta Higgs, and the social services Child Abuse Consultant, Sue Richardson — particularly came in for criticism from hostile professionals, parents, the public, MPs and the media. Many people did not wish to accept that child sexual abuse could be so widespread, and painful issues about the infringement of *parents'* rights were raised.

It is interesting to note that the Cleveland Inquiry Panel reported that, prior to Dr Higgs's appointment in 1987, 'In Cleveland during 1985 and 1986 a number of people had been expressing concern about the response of agencies to child sexual abuse, notably a nursing officer responsible for dealing with abuse in South Tees' (Butler-Sloss, 1988). The Inquiry Report indicates the role played by the

nursing professions in the 'affair'. That involvement includes identifying children who may be at risk: 'In early April, a 3 year old girl
was brought to the Accident and Emergency Department because a
school nurse had noticed excessive bruising' which was felt to indicate
sexual abuse. Commenting on the number of children who had
allegedly been sexually abused and who were admitted to hospital, the
Panel said: 'Most of the children had no medical problem requiring
nursing or medical attention and their presence on the ward caused
difficulties for the nurses.' Surprisingly, however, the Panel made no
specific recommendations concerning nursing practice in the wake of
the events in Cleveland, even though proposals were made regarding
the police, the medical profession, social services, parents, and
children themselves.

The 'discovery' of child abuse in nursing practice

While nursing practice throughout its history has been concerned
with humanistic principles of care, which relate to what has later
become known as child protection, this area of work was not
recognised as such in official guidance to nurses until comparatively
recently. For example, a standard health visiting text in the 1950s by
Margaret McEwan (1959) makes *no* mention of child abuse. However,
there is a chapter entitled 'The Abnormal Family' in which she writes:

> in spite of every effort, there remains a hard core of families which
> include individuals who might be said to have two main character-
> istics: (1) intractable ineducability and (2) instability and infirmity
> of character. (p. 59)

The prevailing view is clearly that of the individual inadequacies
rather than one of broader social structural influences, including the
social position of children.

The early child abuse inquiry reports also make little reference to
or specific recommendations relating to the role of the nursing
profession, even though health visitors and nurses were involved in
most of the cases. The panel inquiring into the death of Maria Colwell
in 1973 identified the role of health professionals and reported:

> the part played by the GP in this particular case cannot be
> regarded as central. Nonetheless . . . GP's are key people in the
> detection of children at physical risk . . . In 1972 it was common
> practice to link the health visitors, employed by local authorities,
> to general practice and this brought this area of the medical
> services into even closer relationships with the social services than
> previously. With the reorganisation of the National Health

Service the structural link has changed. (Department of Health
and Social Security, 1975)

Although the potential for nurses in child protection is noted, this is
not developed.

In 1975 the Department of Health and Social Security held, for the
first time, a day conference on non-accidental injury, the purpose of
which was not just to highlight 'the reality of the threat of violence to
the child in his home, but also the number of professionals concerned
with it and the imperative need for co-ordination between them'
(1975). The report of the conference refers to the prevention of non-
accidental injury and suggests that this is an issue which should also be
addressed by the maternal and child care services, including health
visiting and nursing. One chapter of the report of the day's
proceedings, written by a senior health visitor, states that the health
visitor is integral to child protection work, and there is, for the first
time, a documented discussion of the need for procedural systems for
health visitors working with children 'at risk'.

Since the mid-1970s the work of the nursing professions in the
protection of children has been formally recognised in the various
government guidelines. Partly as a result of the increasing numbers of
child sexual abuse registrations, the then Department of Health and
Social Security asked its Standing Nursing and Midwifery Advisory
Committee to consider the implications of child abuse for the
profession. This led to a consideration of the work of 'senior nurses
who, in the course of their duties, supervise and assist in the training
of practitioners in matters relating to child abuse, including child
sexual abuse' (Department of Health and Social Security, 1988). In
the foreword to the Committee's report, its chair, Suzanne Mowat,
notes:

the circumstances in which children's deaths have occurred over
the past years have demonstrated certain recurring characteristics
in the management arrangements for all practitioners, but particularly for health visitors and school nurses. These characteristics
include uncertainty about incident reporting, confusion about
case conference outcomes and review decisions; and inadequate
monitoring of incidents and concerns. (1988)

It is significant that these topics were identified since they remain
symptomatic of the problems and dilemmas which nurses still face.
Mowat then goes on to say that the working group 'identified a
paramount need for nurses, midwives and health visitors to have
ready access to a senior nurse, or midwife, who is knowledgeable and
experienced in the subject of child abuse'. Thus each health authority
had for the first time to identify a named senior nurse to co-ordinate

nursing work in child protection. Effective nurse management of child protection is very important, but it is interesting that commensurate central guidance has not been offered to the nurses who are providing that care. It is also significant that the underlying causes of the dilemmas faced by nurses in child protection work are not discussed. Instead emphasis is placed on information systems and procedures, without acknowledging the broader social context and the fact that, even though systems have been in place in the past, they have not always worked despite the best intentions of the staff operating them.

Thus, for example, the report comments on the uniqueness of the health visitor's role, which derives from the fact that she offers a universal service, and notes that the health visitor is able to identify 'deviation from the normal in both health and relationship terms' and is thus well placed to recognise the need for action and initiate it at an early stage. There is no discussion in the report about what might be barriers to taking protective action. Instead it is suggested that the senior nurse should establish various systems, including: a communication system with social services and other agencies, such as Family Practitioner Committees; caseload reviews with staff; a system of formal notification of case conferences; an effective system for handover from midwife to health visitor to school nurse; and appropriate systems for record-keeping and reporting.

The importance of these points is not denied — and, indeed, it is a cause for concern that such systems are not always fully implemented or understood; nevertheless, unless the underlying reasons for needing these systems are addressed, nurses will continue to be placed in positions of vulnerability and children placed at risk.

This is perhaps borne out by the fact that, despite the exhortations to set up improved systems of child protection made by different panels of inquiry, which are now almost ritualistically set up following the death of a child, the tragedies continue. The procedures and systems have changed over the years — usually in response to a 'crisis' — but the conflicts and contradictions largely remain unresolved.

Towards resolving the conflicts?

Key Issues in Child Protection seeks to provide a context for the discussion of child protection work in nursing practice and addresses some of the inherent dilemmas which relate, for example, to gender, race, status, professional autonomy and social structure — in short, issues of power. These issues are not widely spoken about in nursing practice in relation to child protection and certainly never find their way into the official guidance. In part this may because they are perceived as being outside the control of managers and individual practitioners. That is short-sighted and nursing practice is the poorer for it.

Women provide the bulk of child care in the family and also comprise the very great majority of the nursing workforce, so gender is a recurring theme throughout this book. Ben Thomas discusses gender in child protection work both from the engendered construction of child abuse and the part played by gender in relationships between professinal workers. He looks at recent developments in the study of gender and applies them to patterns of parenting and to how professionals relate both to parents and to other professionals.

Thomas notes that it is usually only when gender is identified as a problem associated with child abuse that people become aware of its relevance, despite the fact that it can be a significant variable of good practice in all settings. Formal child protection procedures centre, in large part, around the case conference. Thomas comments that women, because of their socially inferior position, can find it difficult to assert themselves and disagree with powerful men around the case conference table. And yet it is often the female health visitor who will know more about the family in question than many of the other professionals participating in the conference. Thomas concludes by highlighting the important role which all professionals have in challenging gender stereotypes.

Race can also be a challenge to effective and appropriate child protection. An anti-racist perspective for child protection has still to be widely adopted, and in the main it is still white ethnocentric values which inform child protection work and workers from all disciplines are predominantly white. Tom Narducci discusses the cultural determinants of child abuse and shows how behaviour is in part labelled to be abusive according to the culture in which it occurs. In addition stereotyped attitudes and a failure to understand the culture of a group may lead professionals to reach wrong conclusions about how that group cares for children. This poses dilemmas for professionals. Certain actions, however, are abusive regardless of the cultural boundaries, and intervention with the family is necessary in order to protect the children. Living and working in a wider society, child protection professionals are as influenced by racist attitudes as anyone else and most of us will recognise racist attitudes within ourselves. There is, moreover, a number of ways in which the practice used by white people can support racism while not being racist in itself. For example, one common approach is 'colour blindness', in which the experience of being black is denied and undervalued by treating the individual as white. Narducci outlines strategies for tackling such issues. He also identifies the need to recognise the danger that professionals, in seeking to be anti-racist, may overlook the abuse of a child simply to avoid being seen as a racist. We all need to question our values in order that we can challenge racist practice whenever it presents and in whatever form.

As we have shown, the rights of parents have been a crucial factor in the construction of child abuse. For many years — and arguably to some degree today — children were seen as the property of their parents, and care-givers and the children could therefore be treated however the parents thought appropriate and that included physical chastisement. Intervention in family life has long been resented and seen as an infringement of parents' liberty. There is a fine line between parents' rights and those of children. The Children Act and the United Nations Convention on the Rights of the Child (UN, 1990) seek to promote the rights of children while at the same time attempting to balance parents' rights. In many respects these are policies which now need to be translated into practice. A children's rights perspective must underpin all child protection work if we are to be truly sensitive to the needs of children and young people. By no means all professionals accept that children have equal rights with parents.

Robyn Pound looks at the prevention of child abuse, but not through the more usual premise of simply identifying vulnerable families who may become 'at risk'. Instead her starting point is the social status of children, their rights as individuals and especially their right to protection from *any* violence in the family, including smacking. In particular she looks at the campaign to end the physical punishment of children. She considers how such civil legislative reform could help nurses, parents and children and, importantly, prevent child abuse.

The debate on making smacking and corporal punishment unlawful has attracted considerable controversy in recent years. Such punishment is now outlawed in many settings — state schools, residential homes and foster care, for example — and yet the law still allows parents to physically punish their children. Many parents feel they have an absolute right to so punish their children, in much the same way that parents in the nineteenth century felt they could treat their offspring exactly as they wished. The EPOCH campaign and its supporters, which include many child care agencies — such as the NSPCC, Save the Children and ChildLine — and professional associations — such as the Health Visitors Association — believe that smacking is damaging, ineffective and, importantly, a denial of children's rights. There is also concern that smacking can escalate into even more damaging forms of abuse as parents lose control, the smack becomes ineffective as a form of discipline — as it always is — and the threshold of what is an acceptable form of punishment is lowered.

A change in civil law to make physical punishment illegal would have a symbolic value, as has been the case with equal opportunities legislation, and certainly the experience of some countries where it has been made illegal is that the incidence of smacking has declined. Public education, however, on the unacceptability of smacking and on positive forms of discipline is crucially important if the behaviour of the majority of parents is to change. However, at the same time, professionals need to work alongside parents, which is not necessarily easy if and when professionals are promoting ideas which are at variance with popular thinking. In seeking to change attitudes the professionals need to work in partnership with the parents and carers.

The concept and practice of partnership in nursing and child protection work is taken up by Carole Peall. 'Working in partnership' is a term much in vogue in the 1990s, but very little thought has actually gone into what this might mean for professional practice. Naish (1992) has pointed to some of the issues for health professionals. The Children Act and *Working Together* guidelines correctly place strong emphasis on children's and parents' rights to participate in decisions affecting their lives. The theory is easier than the practice, and it is all too easy for professionals to pay only lip service to the concepts of partnership.

Peall uses the example of parental attendance at child protection case conferences to illustrate the challenges of working in partnership with parents and children, although the underlying themes will apply to a range of situations. She seeks to demonstrate how professional power can be exerted at a time when parents and children are particularly vulnerable and when the professionals, who also feel vulnerable, have a need to assert a position to justify their actions and recommendations. There is also an imposed dominance of professional overlay knowledge underpinning the interactions. If the principles of partnership and participation are to be effectively put into operation — rather than the 'real business', for example, being conducted outside of the case conference, in the corridors, out of earshot of the parents — then the ambivalent attitudes, fears and difficulties of the practitioners need to be openly addressed and this latter process mandated by the employing organisation. It is difficult to unpack these issues since they will reveal the pratitioner's vulnerabilities in the need to be totally honest. Ironically, it will also be shown that practitioners have in fact a lot in common with the families with whom they are working. This is a positive position from which to build and is a starting point which should be considered in supervision.

Dingwall et al. (1981) have noted that there is much less propensity for therapeutic supervision of child abuse work in nursing practice than in social work. Jane Parkinson builds on this theme and unravels the different meanings and functions of supervision and considers their different applications for the nursing role in child protection. Management, supervision and support can all have different meanings, and it may be possible for the nurse to receive only some of these from her manager. The traditional community nurse's method of working, with an emphasis on individual professional autonomy, may make supervision and support difficult, and it can be left to the nurse to bring identified 'problems' to her manager. Parkinson's arguments are based in part on the research conducted in the health authority where she was employed as a senior nurse in child protection. Parkinson raises important points about whether line managers can meet the supervision and support needs of community nursing staff who are working with abusive families and whether, in any case, a line manager can provide a safe environment in which to discuss feelings about child abuse.

The resource implications of appropriate and effective supervision need to be addressed, and it is a cause for concern that these costs are often not accorded sufficient priority. For the families with whom community nurses are working these costs are not a luxury which can be dispensed with. This debate about supervision in community nursing in relation to child protection is long overdue.

When and how to take decisive action is a recurring theme in the literature of child protection. We have already seen the impact that gender and power relationships have on nursing practice in relation to child protection. Peter Tattersall takes up these issues and offers practical guidance on assertiveness. Tattersall defines what is meant by assertiveness and then goes on to describe why it is important for safe child protection practice. He points out that common overall responses in child protection are ones of either denial or over-reaction. Professionals may deny there is a real problem when there really is, and as a result they will look for reassurance and confirmation that they have taken the right steps. On the other hand, professionals may over-react to a situation and take more draconian measures than are necessary — they are covering their backs. Clearly such decisions relate to how 'child abuse' is defined and the lack of agreement between the public, families, professionals and policy-makers.

Tattersall encourages practitioners to look at their own practice, review their behaviour, and build on their past successes. He identifies situations in which communication can be difficult: giving praise; accepting praise; stating an unpopular opinion; listening to and exploring an unpopular opinion; raising difficulties; responding to criticism; saying 'no'. There are many other examples, but the principles of assertive communication will apply to many situations.

There are many nursing situations in which assertive communication will be of benefit. One such example is when a child presents in an accident and emergency department: the nurse suspects the child may have been abused but the evidence is ambiguous and, in any case, the nurse may feel inexperienced and the department is very busy with many other competing priorities. With whom does the nurse raise her concerns? Is she sufficiently concerned or confident enough to voice her anxieties? Jane Wynne looks at the history of the accident and emergency department in identifying child abuse, the signs and indicators for which to be vigilant, and the actions which should be taken. It is often the nurse who will have most contact with the young patient and whoever brings her into the accident and emergency department, so she may therefore be better placed than the medical staff to assess the overall situation. Jane Wynne considers the issues.

Recent years have seen social workers become identified as the lead profession for responding to child abuse. The nature of social work and their keyworker position has meant that social workers have probably spent more time than other professional groups in thinking about both the professional and personal issues of responding to identified child abuse. There are lessons which can be shared, and Jim Waters seeks to do that, drawing on both his own experience as a social worker and on a project he managed in which health visitors were seconded to work within a specialist child protection team of social workers. Waters explores the supposed polarities of prevention and treatment — or what he calls 'protection' — in responding to the needs of children and their families. He suggests that the confidence of health visitors is sometimes lost between these polarities. Our response to child abuse is increasingly in terms of investigation and assessment, leaving the preventive, supportive and healing aspects underdeveloped.

Waters suggests that, traditionally, health visitors have been most concerned with the preventive end of the continuum and social workers with the treatment end. Both disciplines encounter uncertainties when they move away from the traditional focus of their work, and yet each professional discipline has a lot to offer the other. There is much to commend in the teamwork approach, but the traditional model of health visiting does not necessarily lend itself easily to working in this way. Waters suggests a number of strategies, derived from social work, which may be helpful to health visitors and nurses in their child protection work.

Child protection in the 1990s is dominated by two key documents: the Children Act and the government guidelines *Working Together*. Professionals from all disciplines working with children, including nurses, need to understand the basis, provisions and implications of the Act. Wendy Stainton Rogers and Jeremy Roche outline the philosophy and main contents of the Act. The Act has a number of general and specific implications for health visitors and nurses and provides a broad framework in which the needs of children should be met. In addition there are particular measures which will impact upon specific nursing practice — for example, with regard to the new provisions for parental responsibility, nurses' record-keeping systems will need to be updated to take account of those people who now have parental responsibility. The Act's support for preventive work endorses the work of health visitors and this should mean that they are fully acknowledged as key players in child protection work.

Stainton Rogers and Roche point out that the Act represents a change in philosophy which is in tune with that of nurses and health visitors giving emphasis to a holistic view of the child's welfare and wellbeing, including the vital importance of the child's family, community and identity. The Act also promotes the ideal of working in partnership with families.

The Children Act was implemented in law from October 1991, but it is too soon to say conclusively what has been its real impact. There are, however, tremendous resource and training implications, and many agencies are concerned that the Act's provisions will founder because of a shortage of resources which authorities largely have to find from within their existing budgets. There are very real worries that the preventive measures contained in the Act, which command widespread support, will not be fully implemented. If actual service provision falls short of the ideal set in law, the child protection worker's dilemmas will be aggravated further.

In summary, then, child protection work is based upon a set of highly complex and interlinked social processes and structures. The issues which this book addresses are all fundamentally concerned with the question of power. They are deeply rooted in society and exert a strong and subtle influence on all areas of social life, including nursing practice. Nurses alone, either as individuals or as a profession, cannot resolve this impact on child protection.

However, a recognition and understanding of the links between these issues and nursing practice is an important first step. This will enable the development of critical and reflective practice with the aim of empowering practitioners *and* the children and the families with whom they work.

Nurses can begin to address these issues by discussion and planning together, perhaps facilitated by the various professional associations, and also by discussion with child protection workers from other disciplines. These groups may also provide mutual support. From such initiatives strategies for minimising the impact of power relations on nursing practice may be developed. The development of a collective consciousness, among the family of nursing, of the profound consequences of these factors will do much to improve the effectiveness of child protection.

As a matter of urgency, high on the agenda of discussions by nurses in their different forums must be an analysis of the proper funding of child protection work, since the current levels of resourcing in many areas — as exemplified by shortages of health visitors and the numbers of children placed on child protection registers and not allocated to social workers — leaves children at risk and further disempowers the professionals to whom society gives the important job of protecting children. Child protection workers can and must appraise their practices and beliefs and should be given the time and space to do so, but, if insufficient resources are channelled into these vital services, professionals will continue to struggle to meet need, and the children's basic right to protection from abuse and exploitation will never become universal.

References

Aries, P. (1962) *Centuries of Childhood*. London: Penguin.

Butler-Sloss, E. (1988) *The Report of the Inquiry into Child Abuse in Cleveland 1987*. London: HMSO.

Cook, A., James, J. and Leach, P. (1991) *Positively No Smacking*. London: Health Visitors Association.

Creighton, S. J. (1992) *Trends in Child Abuse*. London: National Society for the Prevention of Cruelty to Children.

Department of Health (1991a) *A Study of Inquiry Reports*. London: HMSO.

Department of Health (1991b) *Children and Young Persons on Child Protection Registers Year Ending 31 March 1990 England*. London: Department of Health.

Department of Health (1991c) *Working Together under the Children Act 1989*. London: HMSO.

Department of Health and Social Security (1975) *Report of the Committee of Inquiry into the Care and Supervision Provided in Relation to Maria Colwell*. London: HMSO.

Department of Health and Social Security (1975) *Non Accidental Injury of Children*. London: HMSO.

Department of Health and Social Security (1988) *Child Protection: Guidance for Senior Nurses, Health Visitors and Midwives*. London: HMSO.

Dingwall, R., Eekelaar, J. and Murray, T. (1981) *Care or Control? Decision-Making in the Care of Children Thought to have been Abused or Neglected*. Oxford: SSRC Centre for Socio-Legal Studies, Wolfson College.

Ferguson, H. (1991) Rethinking child protection practices: a case for history. In The Violence Against Children Study Group, *Taking Child Abuse Seriously*. London: Unwin Hyman.

Finkelhor, D. (1979) *Sexually Abused Children*. New York: Free Press.

Kempe, H. et al. (1962) The battered child syndrome. *Journal of the American Medical Association*, 181, pp. 17–22.

Lambeth, Lewisham, and Southwark Area Review Committee (1989) *The Doreen Aston Report*. London: London Borough of Lewisham.

Levy, A. and Kahan, B. (1991) *The Pindown Experience and the Protection of Children: The Report of the Staffordshire Child Care Inquiry*. Stafford: Staffordshire County Council.

McEwan, M. (1959) *Health Visiting: A Textbook for Health Visitor Students*. London: Faber and Faber.

Naish, J. (1992) Working in partnership. *Journal of the British Association of Child Health*, Summer 1992, p. 3.

O'Toole, R., Turbett, P. and Nalepka, C. (1983) Theories, professional knowledge and diagnosis of child abuse. In Finkelhor, D., Gelles, R., Hotaling, G., and Straus, M., (eds) *The Darkside of Families*. New York: Sage.

Parton, N. (1990) Taking child abuse seriously. In The Violence Against Children Study Group, *Taking Child Abuse Seriously*. London: Unwin Hyman.

United Nations (1990) *Convention on the Rights of the Child*. New York: United Nations.

1 Gender and child protection

Ben Thomas

Gender is a crucial factor in relationships between the caring professionals, particularly health care workers, and their clients, adults or children. The role of gender in cases of abuse has been well analyzed, but the results have been disappointing and have rarely gone beyond equating gender with behavioural differences between the sexes. Likewise, for some time the effect of gender on professionalisation has been widely debated. Such approaches have been criticised owing to their simplistic notion of a taken-for-granted 'sex role theory'. The problem with accepting gender as a 'given entity' means that gender stereotypes and supposed gender-specific attributes are left unchallenged. This is particularly undesirable and in fact detrimental both to clients and professionals in the area of protecting children from abuse, where it is acknowledged that inter-disciplinary and inter-agency work is an essential process.

Inter-disciplinary and inter-agency work calls for trust, openness, understanding and an ability to relate to one another. Gender-stereotyping restricts these abilities and perpetuates divisions and inequality between disciplines. The aim of this chapter is to examine the importance and effect of gender on this particular set of social relations. It examines gender expectations in relation to the professional groups involved in child protection. The chapter is not solely theoretical; it offers guidelines and provides information aimed at assisting health visitors and nurses in the practical aspects of their work.

The meaning of gender

It is commonly accepted that biological sex determines gender, that a natural link exists between male and female anatomy and masculine and feminine behaviours. Bancroft (1989) terms this taken-for-granted view 'anatomical gender'. However, as Savage (1987) argues, the way in which behavioural characteristics are allotted to men or women is a social process, not a natural one. It is often argued that the consequences of ascribing gender role solely to biological causes has resulted in the continued oppression of women by the promotion of a sexual division of labour which is to the advantage of men. While the debate about the extent to which gender roles are socially or innately determined is beyond the bounds of this chapter, attention is given to the cultural view of masculinity and feminity since this view is particularly relevant to parenting, child protection and gender relations at work.

It is often argued that, due to an ascribed role of male breadwin- ner, it is both expected and acceptable for men to be seen as naturally more aggressive than women. Similarly, they are attributed many other 'masculine' qualities such as being competitive, controlling, dominant and performance-orientated. One of the many problems for men of being attributed these characteristics is that many men feel they have to live up to the gender stereotype (Basow, 1986). A second difficulty is that a society which equates masculinity with assertive- ness and encourages and condones men's violence also denies men the opportunity to have, or at least express, other feelings. Looking at all the feelings prohibited to men, we can begin to understand the difficulty many men have relating to people in a meaningful way. After all, what kinds of relationships can be built on the basis of aggressiveness, competitiveness and anger?

Women, on the other hand, are supposedly more passive, subordinate and compliant. Because of their biological adaptation for childbirth and breast-feeding they have become associated with the 'natural' events of child-rearing and domesticity. Women are attri- buted a different set of characteristics based on the idealisation of passivity and condemnation of violence. Segal (1990) suggests that most women from an early age are made aware of obstacles to the expression of their aggression. Unfortunately this may also have negative consequences. Women who disown and repress their anger almost certainly turn their aggressive feelings against themselves or their children.

Gender and parenting

Traditional gender roles, which are reflected constantly in the media and are ingrained in modern society, have been declared to be oppressive to women, resulting in entrapment and leading to child abuse. However, several lines of indirect evidence might lead us to expect that this explanation is too simplistic since gender roles are changing radically. Kimmel (1987) suggests that new role models for men have developed which have not replaced older ones but which have grown alongside them, thereby creating a dynamic tension between ambitious breadwinner and compassionate father. Segal (1990) suggests that most men today desire to have a closer relationship with their children than did their fathers. During the past few years there has been an increase in research into men and masculinity including man's role in the home and workplace.

Historical accounts locate the interest paid to men's involvement in child care and housework in the post Second World War period. Interestingly, the new attention to the father's direct role in child care was first manifested not in research on the quantity or quality of father–child relationships, but rather in studies of what happened when fathers were absent, such as the work of John Bowlby, for example.

Later, during the 1960s, a different emphasis dominated developmental psychology and articulated an influential role for fathers in the development of their children, particularly gender identity (Pleck, 1983). Contemporary child-rearing practices were thought to make it extremely difficult for boys to develop a proper male identity because of initial identification with their mothers and fathers either being absent altogether or unavailable at appropriate times. Allegedly, the combination of too much mothering and inadequate fathering led to insecurity in gender identity for children, especially boys. As this theory evolved, so paternal participation in child-rearing was encouraged. But the new view of the father's role also drew a clear distinction between maternal and paternal roles: mothers have an expressive relationship with both girls and boys, whereas fathers reward male children differently and therefore are the principal transmitters of culturally based conceptions of masculinity and femininity (Biller, 1971).

This more direct but limited role of the father with his children opened the way for a whole new series of studies that considered the influence of fathers on the development and wellbeing of their children. A variety of studies have examined the effects on birth attendance, availability and participation in physical care and play, and the extent to which children model parental behaviour. While many studies demonstrate that men are carrying out more child care and housework than they used to (Simms and Smith, 1982), women still perform the bulk of these tasks, men being more selective in what they choose to do (McKee, 1982; Backett, 1989). As well as being able to provide physical care, many fathers are reported as providing emotional care and support to infants. However, there are few studies which have so far attempted to assess qualitative aspects of the father–child relationship such as perceived closeness.

Shared parenting has been advocated for a number of years, although progress has been slow (Chodorow, 1978). There are obvious impediments to men and women sharing parenting and domestic tasks. The most popular argument is centred around patterns of employment. In Britain two-thirds of married women with children have part-time jobs, and the majority of men with young children work extremely long hours in paid employment (Moss and Brannen, 1987). Whilst men work longest hours outside the home when they have dependent children, the reverse is true of women. It has been reported that married men under thirty with children work four times the amount of overtime as childless men of the same age (Moss and Brannen, 1987). Dual-career families have recently become another area of popular study since they crystallise the contraditions and conflicts provoked when women and men face similar competing demands between work and family. Any equality of sharing in dual-career families has been found to be related to reduction in childcare and housework demands through the hiring of domestic help, usually female, and this is only a solution for the middle classes (Hertz, 1986).

At the other end of the spectrum there is an expectation that the greater involuntary home-centredness of unemployment would lead to increased sharing of child-rearing and domestic tasks between men and women. However, research findings have so far provided a different picture. Both unemployed men and their wives believed more strongly than ever that a man's pride and self-esteem, his sense of masculinity and authority needed to be protected and preserved (McKee and Bell, 1986).

The results from such research finding suggest a very mixed picture. Men do appear to be changing, albeit slowly. However, professionals, particularly those involved in health care, have a major role to play in facilitating this process. The national child professional guidance, *Working Together* (Department of Health, 1991), suggests that during pregnancy and birth, and in the early care of young children, parents are, of necessity, in contact with the maternity and child health services, and this offers opportunities for the preparation and support of parenthood. The overall contribution of medical and nursing staff in this scenario is acknowledged, although major roles will be played by midwives and health visitors. And one of the main recommendations made by Orr (1980) following her interviews with sixty-eight families is that an active policy should be pursued to involve fathers both in the antenatal period and after birth. However, in practice, there still seems little evidence of health visitor involvement or influence with fathers (Meerabeau, 1987).

Direct research into child abuse and parenting has also been increasing. However, these have been for the most part typological studies which have attempted to divide abusing families into types according to common characteristics. A number of common features have emerged from such studies which may be useful in assessing risk and enhancing understanding of the parent. However, the results are derived from small samples, and many of the features identified are not confined to abusing parents. Jones et al. (1987) have produced a scheme for dividing abusing families into smaller groups which is based not only on shared common characteristics, but which has some predictive value in terms of treatment and prognosis. Their suggested typology is based on the initial assessment and eventual outcome of cases in Manchester and Nottinghamshire. According to this model, cases of neglect and injury are based on assessment of a number of factors and then divided into two main groups, primary and secondary abuse, with further subdivisions. An analysis of their 'ideal types' reveals that gender, or rather sex, appears to be an important factor in each case. This, however, is not made explicit, nor is it adequately addressed unless the description of the parent conforms to gender stereotyping, for example, post-natal psychotic mothers and aggressive men with a criminal record of violence.

Consideration of gender in cases of abuse

Considerations of gender are important to all aspects of work related to child protection. Indeed, it could be argued that the very way in which child abuse has been socially constructed and defined in terms of the medical model, with its emphasis on disease and treatment, is gender related (Parton, 1985). The dominant male power over medical practice has resulted in a male rationality of child abuse, making claims based on their own particular interests and views of the world. Parton suggests that this is not only an inadequate explanation but fundamentally misconceived. Consequently, policy and practice has centred on the concept of individual responsibility and on identifying individual patterns of behaviour within particular family relationships. This has deflected attention from the wider issues concerning the social, economic and cultural conditions associated with abuse.

Gender has to be taken into account at all levels, including societal and individual. At an individual level, it is not just the gender of the child or the adult involved in the abuse, but also the gender of the professional worker: the learning that professional workers may have acquired, together with the accumulation of their experiences as women or men, will affect their attitudes and reactions to clients.

However, for the most part it is only when gender or sex becomes identified as a problem that people become aware of its relevance and importance, talk about it, or attempt to deal with it. A few examples from actual case studies demonstrate the point.

A female social worker found it very difficult to work with a young girl who had been physically abused by her father on a number of occasions. The difficulty stemmed from the social worker's intolerance of the child's ambivalence toward the abuser (her father). In exploring this problem with her supervisor the social worker admitted feelings of anger and disappointment towards the child. She could not understand how the child could have any positive feelings towards her father after what he had done to her. With the help of her supervisor, the social worker began to realise that it may not be so irrational for the child to have these feelings. Eventually the social worker began to realise that her own strong negative feelings towards the father, based on a gender stereotype of men as aggressors, was in fact standing in the way of understanding the child's ambivalence and insecurity.

A male community psychiatric nurse (CPN) was party to the disclosure by a female patient of being sexually abused as a child. When he presented the patient's case at a team meeting, some of his female colleagues were outraged at the prospect of him continuing to counsel the woman and suggested that a female nurse from the team should take over the case. In the interest of the patient and against his better judgement he agreed to this plan. Unfortunately the patient took great exception to these arrangements and accused the male CPN of rejecting her and being incapable of handling the information she had disclosed, with the eventual outcome that she refused *any* help offered and left all treatment.

Gender and professional work

Child abuse is a very emotive subject. To most of us, whether public or professionals, it arouses strong feelings, usually feelings of disgust and anger towards the perpetrator, and sympathy and protection towards the child who has been abused. None of us is free from the impact of stereotyping and labelling. Being aware of these feelings whilst not allowing them to impose on our work with clients and patients is a difficult task. Negative attitudes, beliefs and values can interfere with our ability to interview clients, may lead us to produce inaccurate assessments and subsequently affect our decisions and interventions. Clear thinking, emotional control and a non-judgemental approach are essential for the management of abused children and adult offenders.

It is commonly prescribed that for nurses and other health care professionals to provide good practice they must be non-judgemental in their approach to patients and clients. But often as professionals we may be overwhelmed by our own feelings related to the moral, social and legal implications of the case. This may lead us to react in a variety of ways towards the abused child, the parents and others involved in the case. Recent American research which examined the attitudes of 228 professionals to child sexual abuse has clearly demonstrated this point (Parton, 1985). The study subjects included nurses, police officers, teachers, therapists and child protection workers. Results showed that the gender of the child victim influenced the subjects' attitudes towards him or her. The professionals blamed male victims more often than female victims. Male victims were also considered to be at greater risk of becoming homosexuals and offenders as adults. The relationship of the offender to the victim and the social status of the perpetrator also influenced their attitudes. Professionals were much more tolerant of sexual abuse by a child's father than by a non-relative. Offenders with high social status were recommended more lenient prison sentences than those with low social status (Kelley, 1988).

Inter-professional relationships

As in many other areas of human service provision, particularly those involving clinical and social aspects, inter-disciplinary and inter-agency work is an essential process of attempting to protect children from abuse. However, little attention is given to the principles required to enable such a group of professionals to function effectively and efficiently. Managers seem to be under the illusion that simply to bring a group of professionals together in the same room with a common purpose is effort enough to ensure the proper functioning of that team. I acknowledge that each member of the team has a specialist professional contribution to make, but they also have different social backgrounds, training, education and experiences. Often this produces a good cross-section of social classes, ages, races, sexes, attitudes and views. Unfortunately such interplay is not always used as an advantage but rather gives rise to inter-disciplinary rivalry, power struggles and other conflicts leading to poor communication, low morale and ineffectiveness. Sims (1986) describes these problems in terms of various professionals having different interests, priorities, perspectives and language. There is often a lack of respect between disciplines. Negative stereotypical views are held by many professionals, due to their socialisation and training, of the value of other disciplines' contributions. For example, it is often assumed that psychiatrists and social workers have a much more eclectic approach to the causes of human behaviour than police officers who assume that individuals are personally responsible for their behaviour/misbehaviour and who are therefore not interested in societal or psychological contributing factors.

Pollock and West (1984) suggest that judgements of other professionals are affected by gender and sex-role stereotyping and can therefore inhibit team functioning. McIntosh and Dingwall (1978) suggest that among the health care professionals the doctor's dominance is reinforced because of gender and class status, since doctors are often men, and other groups around them women. The prescriptive literature continually emphasises that arrangements for the protection of children from abuse, and in particular case conferences, can only be successful if the professional staff work in partnership and share information (Musanandara, 1984). But there is little research into this important area, particularly in the area of multi-disciplinary decision-taking. There is, however, a growing body of research into the behaviour of professionals in various other small groups. For example, a psychiatric ward round shares many of the characteristics of a case conference (defined as a multi-disciplinary meeting). Research into this area is therefore relevant, although findings need to be interpreted cautiously. An observational study into psychiatric ward rounds demonstrated that most of the time was taken up by discussions on medical and diagnostic issues (Samson Fisher et al., 1979). Medical staff spoke almost eight times as much as non-medical staff, including nurses, and occupational therapists spoke the least.

Sociological literature contains many examples of the silence of one group in the face of another perceived to be more powerful. Pollock (1986) suggests that women find it hard to assert themselves or disagree with powerful men in a team of professionals. Hart (1991) suggests that it is not that nurses do not speak, but that, because what they have to say is not valued by those in power, it is not listened to. Clearly if inter-disciplinary and inter-agency working is to be a reality then it is important for all those involved to be able to contribute and for full consideration to be given to their contribution.

Training

One way to improve the effective functioning of multi-disciplinary teamwork is to provide joint training and to devote time and energy to team building. Multi-disciplinary groups can improve their functioning by joint training in common aspects of their work. In child protection there are many areas which are of mutual concern irrespective of professional boundaries. Examples include recognition of signs of potential abuse, interviewing skills, and legal aspects. Many joint training schemes on child abuse issues have already been implemented. Such programmes are aimed at helping staff from all agencies in the understanding of the respectives roles of the other agencies, and thereby promoting closer working relationships. Training in the area of child sexual abuse has also received increasing attention. The Training Advisory group on Sexually Abused Children (TAGOSAC), in collaboration with the National Children's Bureau, have compiled a database of training resources on child sexual abuse and evaluated their worth (Armstrong and Hollows, 1989).

In addition to training in the areas of skills and knowledge, it is important that issues of gender and sexuality are addressed. These include exploring the different perspectives men and women may have regarding abuse, and the impact of gender at all levels of their work in the protection of children, particularly that related to power. It is *imperative* that the various professionals identify their own values and feelings in order that these do not affect their work adversely. The literature continually illustrates that health care professionals lack knowledge of and comfort with sexual feelings, attitudes, values and beliefs (Webb and Askham, 1987; Thomas, 1989, 1990). This is certainly indicated by my own work in facilitating sexuality workshops for people from a wide variety of disciplines and agencies; despite professionals finding it difficult to cope with many of the areas concerned with gender and sexuality, I have found most are appreciative of the opportunity to do so. It is regrettable that the two major groups noticeable by their absence from such training are male doctors and male police officers.

Team building is often regarded as the most effective intervention for improving inter-disciplinary and inter-agency functioning. The aim of team building is to help those involved analyze how they work together, identify weaknesses, strengths, and make necessary improvements. Team building is particularly useful in addressing issues to do with communication which are often the major obstacles to cohesion, integration and effectiveness.

Conclusion

This chapter has focused on the importance of gender in the area of child protection. It has been argued that considerations of gender are

important to all aspects of child protection. This includes taking
account of the gender of the health care workers and other disciplines
involved in the cases, as well as of those being cared for or otherwise
involved, and the subsequent interactions.

As professionals we have a responsibility to challenge gender
stereotypes wherever they occur and to challenge the limitations
imposed by gender roles, both among our colleagues and in our day-
to-day work with the public.

Parents are responsible for the wellbeing and protection of their
children. It is assumed that child abuse is less likely to happen if there
is an affectionate and positive relationship between parents and child.
Health care workers can do much to encourage parents to take a
responsible attitude to the care of their children, and this must include
fathers. It is important that men are not excluded but are encouraged
to demonstrate affection and are provided with help and support. At
the heart of the problem are our attitudes towards gender stereotypes.
Gender stereotypes must not be taken as given, they must be
challenged and alternatives explored.

References

Armstrong, H. and Hollows, A. (1989) *A Positive Model: Training Papers on Child Sexual Abuse*. London: National Children's Bureau.
Backett, K. (1989) *Mothers and Fathers*. London: Macmillan.
Bancroft, J. (1989) *Human Sexuality and its Problems*. Edinburgh: Churchill Living-stone.
Basow, S. (1986) *Gender Stereotypes: Traditions and Alternatives*. London: Brooks/Cole Publishing Company.
Biller, H. (1971) *Father–Child and Sex Role*. Lexington, MA: Heath.
Chodorow, N. (1978) *The Reproduction of Mothering: Psychoanalysis and the Sociology of Gender*. Berkeley: University of California Press.
Department of Health (1991) *Working Together under the Children Act 1989*. London: HMSO.
Friedson, E. (1977) The future of professionalism. In M. Stackey and M. Reid (eds.), *Health and the Division of Labour*. London: Croom Helm.
Hart, E. (1991) Ghost in the machine. *Health Service Journal*, 5 December, pp. 20–22.
Hertz, R. (1986) *More Equal than Others: Women and Men in Dual Career Marriages*. Berkeley: University of California Press.
Jones, D., Pickett, J., Oates, M. and Barbor, P. (1987) *Understanding Child Abuse*. 2nd edn. London: Macmillan.
Kelley, S. (1988) Professionals' attitudes towards child sexual abuse. *Nursing Times*, 84, p. 56.
Kimmel, M. S. (1987) Rethinking 'masculinity': new directions in research. In M. S. Kimmel (ed.), *Changing Men: New Directions in Research on Men and Masculinity*. Newbury Park: Sage.
McIntosh, J. and Dingwall, R. (1978) Teamwork in theory and practice. In R. Dingwall and J. McIntosh (eds.), *Readings in the Sociology of Nursing*. Edinburgh: Churchill Livingstone.

McKee, L. (1982) Fathers' participation in infant care: a critique. In L. McKee and M. O'Brien (eds.), *The Father Figure*. London: Tavistock.

McKee, L. and Bell, C. (1986) His unemployment, her problem. In S. Allen et al. (eds.), *The Experience of Unemployment*. London: Macmillan.

Meerabeau, L. (1987) Images of fatherhood in antenatal literature. *Health Visitor*, 60, pp. 79–87.

Moss, P. and Brannen, J. (1987) Fathers and employment. In C. Lewis and M. O'Brien (eds.), *Reassessing Fatherhood*. London: Sage.

Musanandara, T. (1984) Communication between workers: the key in cases of child abuse. *Health Visitor*, 57, p. 233.

Orr, J. (1980) *Health Visiting in Focus: A Consumer View of Health Visiting in Northern Ireland*. London: Royal College of Nursing.

Parton, N. (1985) *The Politics of Child Abuse*. London: Macmillan.

Pleck, J. (1983) The theory of male sex identity: its rise and fall, 1936–present. In M. Lewin (ed.), *In the Shadow of the Past: Psychology Views the Sex*. New York: Columbia University Press.

Pollock, L. (1986) The multi-disciplinary team. In C. Hume and I. Pullen (eds.), *Rehabilitation in Psychiatry: An Introductory Handbook*. Edinburgh: Churchill Livingstone.

Pollock, L. and West, E. (1984) On being a woman and a psychiatric nurse. *Senior Nurse*, 1, 17, pp. 10–13.

Samson Fisher, R. W., Poole, A. D. and Harker, J. (1979) Behavioural analysis of ward rounds within a general hospital psychiatric unit. *Behavioural Research and Therapy*, 17, pp. 333–48.

Savage, J. (1987) *Nurses, Gender and Sexuality*. London: Heinemann.

Segal, L. (1990) *Slow Motion: Changing Masculinities, Changing Men*. London: Virago Press.

Sims, D. (1968) Inter-organisational: some problems of multi-organisational teams. *Personal Review*, 15, pp. 27–31.

Sims, D. and Smith, C. (1982) Young fathers: attitudes to marriage and family life. In L. McKee and M. O'Brien (eds.), *The Father Figure*. London: Tavistock.

Thomas, B. (1989) Asexual patients. *Nursing Times*, 85, pp. 49–51.

Thomas, B. (1990) Working out sexuality. *Nursing Times*, 86, pp. 41–3.

Webb, C. and Askham, J. (1987) Nurses knowledge and attitudes about sexuality in health care — a review of the literature. *Nurse Education Today*, 7, pp. 75–87.

2 Race, culture and child protection

Tom Narducci

Both the Children Act 1989 and the revised *Working Together* guidelines call upon us in spirit, if not as an actual duty, to give due consideration to the religious persuasion, racial origin and cultural and linguistic background of children with whom we are concerned. In stating that, as in choosing the title for this chapter, there is always the risk that one could identify ethnicity and culture as problems which need to be dealt with rather than issues which need to be addressed. The existence of different ethnic groups, like the existence of various cultures within a dominant culture, is not a problem. Racism, both overt and covert, and racist violence are. It is for that reason too that we no longer refer to 'race awareness training' but to anti-racist or anti-discriminatory training instead. Simply being aware of the existence of other ethnic or cultural groups does not go far enough.

Terms used

Throughout this chapter I use the terms 'ours' and 'we' quite deliberately to denote that it is an exploration of these issues by a white writer, and one which is addressed to members of a mainly white professional group. I shall also refer to ethnicity instead of race. The concept of race is a social construct which has no basis in fact. There is not even agreement, for example, on how many races there are. Ethnicity, however, reflects not only the varied backgrounds but also issues of power which are reflected within society.

More important is the need to clarify how the dominant culture in any society can oppress minority groups, whether intentionally or not, and the effects of that oppression for both victims and perpetrators.

In child protection in particular, we need to be certain that any decisions we make regarding the care or future of any child are based on an objective assessment of facts and not on assumptions or stereotyped views we may hold, unconsciously or otherwise.

Fully understanding the black perspective or experience of being black in Britain today is arguably impossible for white people. In saying that, and in the remainder of this chapter, the term 'black' is used in its widest sense, namely to denote non-white. This reflects an important point since black people will have had a shared experience of which white members of British society cannot have full knowledge. Recognising and acknowledging that shared experience of oppression and discrimination is essential if we, as whites, are to understand both the reason for black people identifying themselves as 'black' and their suspicion of and/or hostility towards white institutions and agencies. White people asked to describe themselves rarely refer to their skin colour. They take their whiteness for granted, as normal, the natural state of affairs, as understood. This lies at the heart of the matter, as it underpins the very foundations of racism, especially in its more insidious forms.

A number of years ago I was introduced to a conceptual model by a black colleague, Bill Sandhu, which is useful in helping to clarify how this process occurs.

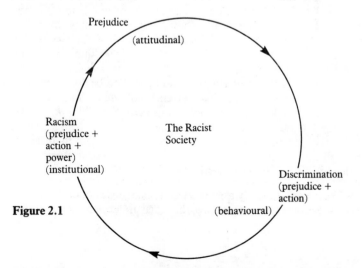

Figure 2.1

Prejudice and institutional racism

Prejudice, that pre-judging based on stereotyped views and assumptions, causes us to believe certain myths and misconceptions regarding ethnic minorities as if they were fact. In turn, this may alter or influence the way we behave towards members of that group. This behavioural component of discrimination then becomes internalised within society and is reflected within the agencies in that society. That institutional racism both legitimises and reinforces the holding of those prejudices, and so the cycle continues. It is also the basis of those economic differentials and inequalities apparent in comparisons of achievement levels of black and white people. In relation to child care issues, it should be remembered that we place expectations on black parents of providing certain standards while denying them a fair chance at achieving that possibility.

Many white readers will say 'Yes, I recognise that risk but know that it doesn't pertain to me or to the way I work with black families and children'. My argument is simply that unless we confront these issues and genuinely look at our own attitudes and beliefs, then non-discriminatory practice cannot be guaranteed. 'The black child may not just be a victim of abuse, or at risk. She or he may be the victim of ignorance, dilemma, unawareness, subjective judgement, insensitivity and prejudice of the social work (and other) professions. She or he may be at the receiving end of personal and institutional racism' (Ahmad, 1989). If any of us takes a few moments to consider privately all the negative comments we can remember having heard both as a child and as an adult regarding members of different ethnic or cultural groups, can we be totally certain that we have not internalised any of those within our own belief system?

Assuming that there is within each of us some aspect of racist belief, this then necessitates an examination of our behaviour and practice in order to determine how, not if, we may in reality discriminate against not only the black consumers of our services but also our black colleagues. Overt racists, I have little doubt, will either not read this chapter or simply dismiss its contents. I shall concentrate instead on how those of us who would not wish to be discriminatory may, through our behaviour, inadvertently collude with racism.

Lena Dominelli, in her book *Anti-racist Social Work*, (1988) highlighted a number of strategies used by white people which endorse racism while at the same time not being racist in themselves. Although there is clearly some overlap between these strategies, it is worth exploring each of them briefly:

- *omission* — simply assumes that racism does not exist. Race is irrelevant as are, therefore, the racial dimensions of any and all social interactions.

- *denial* — we fail to acknowledge racism in both ourselves and society. We think of it as the personal prejudices and behaviours of a few extreme and irrational individuals but refuse to accept the existence of cultural and institutional racism.
- *decontextualisation* — means accepting the existence of racism but not recognising or accepting its permeation into day-to-day routines. Racism is something 'out there' somewhere but does not affect the day-to-day lives of our patients or clients.
- *dumping* — the assigning of black workers to work with black families or getting black trainers to do the training. Using this method we give black people, the victims of racism, the responsibility for getting rid of it and whites carry on as usual.
- *colour blindness* — appears to be a fairly common method. We negate black people's experience of being black by treating them as if they were white. We ignore their discrimination by denying their reality.
- *patronising* — in this strategy black people are tolerated as some aberration from the norm. White values are deemed to be superior, thereby underlying the basis of institutional racism since comparisons of, for example, child-rearing practices will be made against those considered to be 'normal' (white).
- *avoidance* — simply avoiding confronting issues, for example by hearing racist comments, feeling uncomfortable but staying silent. This occurs particularly when the comment is made by someone with authority and power.

It is not, I would guess, difficult for any of us to recognise examples of when we have ourselves used one of the above strategies in either our personal or professional lives. But not only do these strategies collude with racism, they also affect both the service we offer to patients and clients and the way it is perceived. Carol Baxter highlights how simple it is for these strategies to interfere with the development of that relationship:

> It is [equally] important that all health and social welfare professionals work at developing a relationship of mutual respect and trust and demonstrate to black and ethnic minority families that their discretion and child rearing methods are not being judged as deficient or inferior. (Baxter, 1989)

If we do not respect their reality, are not willing to trust, and judge their child-rearing methods as deficient or inferior to our own, then how are we to offer either an appropriate or relevant service to those families, and why should they perceive us as their ally?

Culture and child protection

Turning from the issue of ethnicity to that of culture presents us with the immediate problem of defining what we mean by the term. From conversations and through training sessions held around the country, it is clear to me that many people use these concepts as if they mean the same thing. While this is, and can be, true of a small number of cultures whose members all share an ethnic heritage, it is clearly not true of the majority of the population. Culture is defined in *Collins Concise English Dictionary* as 'the total of the inherited ideas, beliefs, values and knowledge which constitute the shared basis of social action'. But what does that mean to us, and specifically in relation to issues in the area of child protection? Korbin has written:

> Dealing with child abuse and neglect is difficult enough within a community sharing a basic definition of abuse. The problem is exacerbated when different communities come into contact, or when sub-cultural groups, often referred to as communities in their own right, differ in their beliefs about child rearing practices including child abuse and neglect. (Korbin, 1979)

What this means in effect is that what is perceived as abusive or neglectful within one culture may not be viewed in the same light in others. For example, Polynesian mothers view the western practice of infants being put in separate beds in separate rooms as detrimental to child development and potentially dangerous, whereas I can clearly recall discussions between professionals and young mothers warning them of the dangers of letting a new-born infant sleep in the same bed as themselves in case the child should accidentally be suffocated. Think too, of the cases in which there has been a fear of potential abuse due to the 'battle of wills' between a carer and child in the area of toilet training. Jill Korbin makes the point that, while this is clearly an area of stress and potential risk in western cultures, it is not always considered to be so in others, since their starting point is an assumption that the child will toilet itself when necessary and in the appropriate area once the child has the physical maturity to control these functions.

A number of decisions regarding child care and child protection are made on an almost daily basis in this country, and we must ask ourselves how many of these are made in accordance with judgements about the inappropriateness of others' cultural practices as compared with our own white British practice. Within the African-Caribbean community, for example, a number of family 'models' operate, one of which is the grandmother–mother–child model. Marriage is often delayed until economic security is ensured, leading to a stereotyping

of black women as 'single parents'. This is clearly not the case and is
based on a misunderstanding of a culturally accepted model, since in
reality there are more white single mothers than black in the UK.
There is, however, no stereotyping of white families as mainly single-
parent families (Anonymous).

Working with members of other cultural groups can become
further complicated if we attribute to them belief systems based on
our own. The report of the Popular Project highlights some of the
difficulties this assumption can cause (London Borough of Tower
Hamlets Social Services Department, 1991). The case involved a
number of Bangledeshi boys who had been sexually abused, and
during the investigation and the follow-up work staff became aware of
a number of major difficulties caused through making that assumption. Most of the boys involved came from Muslim families, and
within Muslim society there are clear guidelines as to what is and is not
allowed to be openly discussed. Questions of sexuality and sexual
activity are not open for discussion outside of the family and certainly
not with children. The report also highlighted the difficulties
surrounding the issue of language. There are no equivalent terms in
the Bengali language to describe sexual abuse. This led to a situation
which involved the staff having to imply that sexual abuse had
occurred by referring to a 'bad thing' having happened, followed by
crude descriptive details of the actual abuse itself.

This raises further questions, some of which were recognised in
the report itself, but especially as to whether we aim to provide an
ethnically and culturally sensitive service or merely impose western
values on people living in this country. While I am not suggesting for
a moment that the above case did not need to be investigated and the
boys and their families offered help, it does raise questions as to what
approach we take and what help we can offer when our starting points
are so different. Perhaps we need to begin by not assuming that one
single approach is enough.

Respect for culture and protection — a dilemma?

As I stated at the beginning of this chapter, recent government
guidelines and legislation regarding child protection require us to
consider the cultural background of families with whom we are
working. This can, however, leave us with what feels like a basic
dilemma when attempting to achieve a balance between respecting
people's cultures and protecting children. African-Caribbean parents, for example, are sometimes said to be over-strict. However, a
number of black colleagues have argued that for 'over-strict' we

should substitute 'protective and caring', since the black parents' concern as to whether their child behaved well in school or where their teenage son was in the evening could also be seen as a reflection of their recognition that their child will need higher school results and is more likely to be stopped by the police if on the streets at night. Criticisms are made too regarding parenting that involves the shared care of children by the extended family. This has often been identified as a dumping of responsibility and as failing to provide children with either continuity or stability.

It was, however, the model previously practised in this country within the indigenous culture and is clearly still the preferred model in a number of cultures around the world. Far from a dumping of any sort, it is seen as a way of both supporting young families and offering the children additional stimulation and developmental opportunities. It simply depends on how you choose to look at it.

In observations of some Asian and other cultures, daughters have been seen as being pushed into stereotyped roles as the assistant and pupil to the mother. Judgements are made that the child has been placed in an unhappy role based on outdated gender-stereotypes. This is a view based on a value judgement made against what we consider to be normal activity for adolescent girls. Perhaps more seriously, Melody Mtezuka makes the point that 'western observers could be forgiven for suspecting that the role taken by the female child was extended to include sexual behaviour. Writers such as Finkelhor and Waterman comment on such behaviour as indicative of sexual abuse' (Mtezuka, 1990). This is an important point, since some of the current work and certain theories about child sexual abuse revolve around the basic premise of the daughter becoming a substitute for the wife. But this premise needs to be challenged when working with those from a culture which does not view that role as either exploitative or as a prelude to abuse. Traditional cultural values, although perhaps not to our liking, should not be judged as abusive.

As can be seen, when considering the question of culture and child protection, we need to address a number of questions before deciding what, if any, action should be taken and if so, how. Having clarified what we mean by culture, our next step should be to ask ourselves why we should respect other people's cultures within Britain. Should they not, having decided to move here, adopt 'British culture' as their way of life? Much has been written on this subject. Both the model and strategies offered earlier are again useful since they help us to understand how simple it becomes to judge other cultures against our own, on the basis that 'ours' is superior to 'theirs'. Different should not mean inferior. Holding those views would also negate the value and dynamism added to British culture through integrating aspects of others into its thinking and beliefs.

When is intervention appropriate?

Having said that, it is clearly right that children from minority ethnic groups and cultures should be protected, a point I shall return to later. However, at this point we need to confront the question of when it is right to intervene and set aside other people's cultural beliefs. Clearly there are cases where particular practices, although possibly culturally acceptable in another place, are not acceptable in the United Kingdom in the 1990s. The most obvious example of this is female circumcision. The Prohibition of Female Circumcision Act 1985 'makes female circumcision, excision and infibulation (female genital mutilation) an offence except on specific physical and mental health grounds' (Department of Health, 1991).

The law can and does protect children from what are seen as extreme practices; however, we should be clear that there are no identified cultures in which child abuse or neglect are condoned. There are case examples where schoolteachers and other professionals suspecting sexual abuse of children from minority ethnic cultures, questioned whether this was culturally the norm and therefore not open to the same challenge. There are no cultures which sanction child sexual abuse.

One last question regarding culture needs to be addressed and that is: How, if we decide intervention is necessary, do we help our patients or clients to understand and appreciate why we have acted as we have? It would be unacceptable to simply intervene in any family without helping, or at least attempting to help, their understanding of our actions, particularly when they may not even understand our initial concern. Should we take that course, we are simply mirroring the worst aspects of institutional racism and cultural dominance as outlined in the conceptual model above. Not only should we not compare or judge other cultural practices against our own white western culture, we should also not use our position of authority to simply enforce our views on others. Action to protect children should be taken, but there is a way of doing this sensitively, and a way of simply doing it based on an abuse of power. Through attempting to assist a family's understanding of us we may also begin to understand them.

We also need to be clear regarding the assumptions we make about the strength and ties within communities and between members of communities and their community leaders. Melody Mtezuka makes the point that 'there was strong criticism of the use of community or religious leaders as intermediaries . . . If confidentiality was important in working with white families it was equally important for Asian families' (Metzuka, 1990).

Without denying the potential role of church and community

leaders in responding to child abuse, there are rare exceptions within
child protection procedures and practice where church or community
leaders are given access to information regarding the possibility or
actual abuse of children within a particular family. It is felt to be a
matter between the professionals and the family, and we should not
make assumptions that members of ethnic and cultural minority
families would be happy or expect us to involve their community or
religious leaders in their affairs.

It may well be appropriate, with the approval of the family, to seek
support from the community at some stage in the future. It is clearly
not appropriate to approach members of the community, whether
they be religious leaders or not, with a view to gaining information
about a family as part of an investigation or assessment without their
expressed consent. They may be the last people the family would wish
to know their business.

A shared responsibility

It may seem that, in attempting to be sensitive to ethnic and cultural
issues, we create for ourselves difficulties which until now were not
difficulties at all. I said earlier that it was clearly not the sole
responsibility of our black colleagues to address these issues, and
equally it is important we acknowledge it is not the sole responsibility
of our black colleagues to either work with all black families or
suddenly become our 'experts' on issues to do with ethnicity and
culture. There is a responsibility on all of us to offer a service to
children and families within the community at large which is both
relevant and appropriate to their needs. We need to ensure that
children from these minority ethnic groups are afforded the same
protection and have their rights to be free from harm or neglect
respected. Black colleagues can clearly help us in this by supporting
one another to challenge assumptions and stereotypes as well as
examples of other poor practices related to management issues. As
members of some of these minority ethnic groups, they are clearly in
a position to help us too to understand various aspects related to those
groups. However, we should remember that as we are not in a position
to speak on behalf of all white people, neither are our black colleagues
in a position to speak on behalf of all of those black people living in
Britain today. There are clear differences of history, religion,
language and cultural background which would exclude their having
any more knowledge of a particular group than anyone else outside
that group.

We should not forget that, through 'openly and positively
addressing racial and cultural differences' (Thomas, 1989), we open

ourselves to a better communication between ourselves, our colleagues and the families with whom we work. Through recognising the limits of our knowledge, we acquire the opportunity for our work to be a learning and enriching experience too. We would not claim to be aware of all there is to know regarding the pressures of everyday life felt by white British families, and neither should we be afraid to recognise and to admit that we do not understand all we need to know about families from ethnic and cultural minorities. The dangers are not from not having the knowledge but from making decisions as if we did and from not attempting or believing it necessary to find out. We need to remember too the economic and power differentials which exist. Families exist within a context, and it does neither them or us any service to ignore that context.

Gray, writing with reference to the USA, states:

> The protective services system [in the United States] may be committing a form of institutional abuse of minority families if the professionals that work in that system are not sufficiently well versed in the unique child rearing practices of each culture in the communities this system represents. It is easy for misunderstandings to occur from an ethnocentric perspective, and these misunderstandings are unlikely to be in the minority group's favour. (Gray and Cosgrove, 1985)

If we are to avoid these misunderstandings in the future, and to offer a service which is relevant and appropriate, giving due consideration to the religious persuasion, ethnic origin and cultural and linguistic background of the children with whom we are concerned, then we need to ask and to learn.

We must also recognise there is a danger in our attempting to be anti-racist and culturally sensitive that we may inadvertently overlook the abuse of a child simply to protect ourselves from being labelled as racist. This is equally true for our black colleagues in that they may be challenged, or even feel themselves, that they are turning against one of their own, of being part of a racist system. Being anti-racist and culturally sensitive does not and cannot mean providing a lower level of care and protection to children from these groups. If anything it means the opposite, that these children will be afforded the same care and protection as any other child, but that should something go wrong, then that child and its family will receive a service which is not abusive, irrelevant or based on stereotyped assumptions and prejudices.

I am aware that, for some, reading this chapter may prove to be an overwhelming or paralyzing experience, especially for those who may not have considered some of these issues before. It has sought, through the highlighting of some of the mistakes which can and have been made, to demonstrate how ethnically and ethically poor practice can be avoided and good practice aimed for. Ethnicity and culture should not be seen as problems to be dealt with but as issues to be addressed. That cannot happen overnight but neither can it be left until tomorrow, or worse — to others.

As a starting point, I would suggest each of us should at least

- begin to question the values expressed in our statements and actions. What beliefs underpin them and what are they based upon?
- consider which of the strategies we may be using and how they hinder our developing good working relationships with both our black colleagues and the black consumers of our services.
- begin to challenge judgements made by others of cultural practices when those judgements are based on assumptions and/or on comparisons against our own, rather than on their value in their own right.
- acknowledge we do not always understand and try not to be afraid to ask.

Living in a multi-cultural, multi-ethnic society places a responsibility upon us all but even more so when, as professionals, we are there to provide a service to the community at large. If that service is to be both relevant and appropriate then we need to begin to question not only the way in which we provide it, but also, and more importantly, the values which underpin it.

References

Ahmad, Bandana (1989) Protecting black children from abuse. *Social Work Today*, 20, (39) p 24.
Anonymous *Black Family Life: The Family Must Survive*.
Baxter, Carol (1989) Race and child abuse. *Health Visitors Journal*, 62, 9, pp 271–272.
Department of Health (1991) *Working Together under the Children Act 1989*. London: HMSO, p. 11.
Dominelli, Lena (1988) *Anti-racist social work: a challenge for white practitioners*. Practical social work series. Basingstoke: Macmillan.
Gray, E. and Cosgrove, J. (1985) Ethnocentric perception of child rearing practices in protective services. *Child Abuse and Neglect*, 9 (3) pp. 389–396.
Korbin, Jill (1979) A cross-cultural perspective on the role of the community in child abuse and neglect. *Child Abuse and Neglect*, 3 (1) pp 9–18.
London Borough of Tower Hamlets Social Services Department (1991) *Poplar Project: a social work team's account of its work with a group of sexually abused young people*.
Mtezuka, Melody (1990) Towards a better understanding of child sexual abuse among Asian communities. *Practice Journal*, 3 (3/4) pp 248–260.
Thomas, Greta (1989) Points for consideration when assessing black children of African and African-Caribbean descent and their families.

3 Promoting positive parenting: new horizons for the prevention of child abuse

Robyn Pound

Why prevention?

In order to prevent the physical and emotional abuse of children, it is necessary to look at the whole of our society and the frequency with which physical punishments and humiliating experiences are common to the majority of children. For most children, it is too late to wait until the signs of child abuse are evident and the family have come under the gaze of professionals. To wait until traces can be recognised and reliably labelled 'abuse' leaves a vast majority of children living in a punitive environment where they may experience emotional and physical damage which, though often not recognised, can have resultant sequelae in later life. The issue of the rights of children is central to the prevention of child abuse; the main aim of primary prevention should therefore be to effect a change in the status of children within our society which at present relegates children to a second-class status. Paramount within this aim is a shift in attitudes which at present allows parents to manage their children's behaviour by using physical punishments. To influence societal attitudes by the gradual diffusion process of health promotion is notoriously slow, especially in this case, when the law still supports parental physical punishment. Legal reform must therefore be part of the process.

The aims of professionals involved in child protection work must therefore be:

- to effect a change in attitudes of individual parents against the use of all physical punishments of children;
- to help parents utilise positive discipline as an alternative to the concept of punishments;
- to effect a change in societal attitudes against the physical punishment of children, including those held by professional workers;
- to actively campaign to change the law, which at present allows parents and others they delegate child care to in the family home to hit children.

By the time child abuse is diagnosed, parenting methods are usually firmly established and often become an adversarial power game which is difficult to change. Parents who have established an authoritarian relationship, possibly requiring escalating force to retain control, may find it very difficult to adopt more co-operative family relationships. The more indulgent parents, who do not provide any clear behaviour boundaries for their children but use physical punishments to regain control, are also likely to find change difficult.

Resistance is understandable in families who feel they have been 'found out' for going too far, when the boundaries of 'too far' are not clearly delineated under the law. Suggestions about change imposed by outside 'experts' can themselves then be seen as punishment, reducing the impact and usefulness of any professional help given. We must begin a programme of preventive child abuse work *before* the establishment of parenting-by-punishment patterns and *before* we identify factors which may put children and their families at risk of abuse.

Smacking in context

Many studies have shown that the majority of UK parents smack their children, and mothers appear to administer most of the day-to-day punishments (Gallup Poll, 1989). The Newson Study in Nottingham (1989) showed that 63 per cent of parents smacked before their child was one year old, and nearly all children have been hit by the age of four — 7 per cent more than once a day, and a further 68 per cent more than once a week. By seven years of age some 22 per cent have been hit with an implement. Interestingly, a quarter of parents from socio-economic groups 1 and 2, composed mainly of professionals and managers, have used an implement by this age, which is a higher percentage than for all parents *in toto*. These findings show the degree to which physical punishment as a method of teaching children how to behave is a norm in our society.

It is a very small percentage of parents who extend physical punishment to serious injuries (Creighton, 1984), an event often related by them to a concept of punishment which has gone 'too far' (Jones et al., 1987). A much larger number of children receive smacks in the name of 'ordinary punishment', as part of everyday parenting, which may well interfere with their mental and physical wellbeing, but do not come to the attention of professionals simply because this method of disciplining children is acceptable in our society. If this norm were shifted so that physical punishments were not an acceptable method of teaching children and fewer parents did it, then the line for 'too far' would become a clear and distinct boundary.

The political context

The human rights movement of this last century has shifted opinion and behaviour on violence. As Peter Newell says:

> Our society has moved away from treating as acceptable the hitting of wives, servants, apprentices; more recently away from acceptance of corporal punishment in the armed forces and judicial corporal punishment; and most recently, away from allowing children to be hit in schools and child care institutions. (1989, p. 13)

Children in the home remain the only section of our society who are not protected from violence under the law. This extension of rights to children has been slow to be realised, as many fear the collapse of parental authority within the family and also have difficulty harmonising the duality of parental rights with children's rights. However, children's rights *have* begun to be placed on the social agenda, although the question of their right to protection from violence in the family home has not, as yet, fully addressed the category of smacking and physical punishment. The United Nation's Convention on the Rights of the Child, adopted by the General Assembly in 1989 and ratified in the UK in December 1991, insists that

> State parties shall take all appropriate legislative, administrative, social and educational measures to protect the child from all forms of physical or mental violence, injury or abuse, neglect or negligent treatment, maltreatment or exploitation, including sexual abuse, while in the care of parent(s), legal guardian(s) or any other person who has care of the child. (Newell, 1991, p. 165)

In the UK the Children Act 1989, which has developed and extended the notion of children as equal citizens, still has not questioned parental use of physical punishments. Those making a case for alternative methods of managing children are largely left unsupported by the law. However, other countries have taken up this issue. In 1979, Sweden became the first country to legally prohibit all physical punishment of children. It was followed by Finland in 1984, Denmark in 1986, Norway in 1987 and Austria in 1989. Nearer to home, the Scottish Law Commission issued a discussion paper in 1990 on parents' rights and responsibilities, which seeks views on whether Scottish parents should lose their right to smack. Things are beginning to change.

What is wrong with physical punishment?

There are good reasons for joining the growing tidal wave of opinion against the use of physical punishment. Research into the short- and long-term effects of child physical punishment is plentiful and persuasive. Evidence from numerous studies shows that repeated physical punishment by parents encourages aggression to persist in their children (Bandura, 1973), creates school bullies, is linked with learning and behavioural problems (Calam and Franchi, 1987), delinquency and possibly even an eventual criminal record (Wolfe, 1987). Social learning theorists suggest that aggression is a learned response to adverse situations (Bandura, 1977), and the extent to which it can be attributed to an innate drive provoked by frustration is a matter for continuing debate (Atkinson et al., 1990). Evidence also clearly illustrates a cycle of aggression; aggressive parents having been handled aggressively by their own parents (Miller, 1987). Adult actions may often speak louder than words, the message to children who are hit being that hitting another person is an acceptable means of settling arguments and differences, especially if you are bigger (Bandura et al., 1973). Eron (1987) concluded that aggressiveness seems to be established during childhood and remains relatively stable thereafter.

Research also shows that the use of physical punishments disturbs the development of moral reasoning and conscience in children. Parents who use explanations and inductive reasoning attain higher rates of compliance and increased moral reasoning in their children than those who rely on power assertion or love withdrawal (Peters, 1981; Baumrind and Black, 1967). Quite simply, children are better behaved because they are more likely to have a well-developed conscience when they understand the reasoning (Wolfe, 1989).

Along the continuum of violence from the tap on a baby to the fatal beating of a child, it is impossible to reach consensus on the degree of force necessary to change physical punishment from being acceptable into not acceptable. A 1990 survey of 76 social services departments in the UK reported that up to half the referred families described their actions as 'ordinary' physical punishment: 'There are relatively few cases of deliberate cruelty and the vast majority of incidents dealt with represent over-chastisement or a loss of control in administering physical punishment' (EPOCH, 1990, p. 97). We need to draw a clear line outlawing *all* physical punishment of children and ensuring parents (and others) know that the risk of damage from escalating violence is not acceptable.

Smacks and threats teach children little about what was wrong in their behaviour, do not allow another point of view and do not offer more acceptable alternatives. Smacks, even little ones, portray aggression and often anger, even if parents say they do it 'for love'. The smack may well lead children to retaliate, so that the incident escalates beyond its original importance, and a legacy of unhappiness and guilt is compounded with each power struggle. Children will integrate these experiences into their self-image and, as Carl Rogers has suggested, the more people are forced to deny their own feelings and accept the values of others, the more uncomfortable they will feel about themselves (Rogers and Stevens, 1967).

Coopersmith (1967) found that children at the ages of ten to twelve years, disciplined by means of physical punishment, were much more likely to have a low self-esteem and manifest deviant behaviour patterns. Feelings of worthlessness and alienation are prevalent amongst adult individuals diagnosed as suffering from mental illness (Atkinson et al., 1990). If poor self-esteem and lack of self-worth is established in childhood, it is likely to persist into adult life. Others have described the link between extreme pathological behaviours in adults, such as the sexual abuse of children and rape, with previous physical punishment (Newell, 1989).

Certainly there are many people who experienced physical and emotional trauma during childhood who appear unscathed in their later life. The degree to which children will be affected by their experience of punishments appears difficult to predict. However, it remains certain that enough are sufficiently affected to warrant public concern. Calam and Franchi found in their study of the consequences of child abuse that the seriousness of injuries did not predict eventual developmental outcome for the child (Calam and Franchi, 1987). Protective factors are difficult to isolate, but may be due to children building a basic trust in themselves and in other people through a sense of being valued as individuals themselves. The availability of a confidant who will offer unconditional reward seems important.

The health promotion role of the community nurse

Community nurses, especially health visitors and school nurses who work with child and family populations, are in a key position to promote positive attitudes towards parenting and an awareness of the rights of children. However, they need first to examine their own values, particularly in relation to the concept of equal rights, something which is not necessariy facilitated within nurse education. For example, research by Jean Orr, which explored the attitudes of student health visitors, found they predominantly held a patriarchal view of society with little awareness of social divisions, let alone any awareness of the degree of sexual inequality (Orr, 1986).

It can be assumed that a considerable number of the nursing profession use smacks on their own children at home. A nurse's practice is constructed by current social values and beliefs, and it is essential that we thoroughly examine our own experiences of childhood and parenting *before* we impose them on our patients/clients. This has obvious implications for nurse education.

It is equally necessary for nurses to understand the context of women who, as mothers, provide most of the child care and mete out the day-to-day punishments. Ong (1986) suggests that the low status and powerless situation of women within a male-dominated public sphere make personal growth a last priority for women as mothers. Their lack of public power is in contradiction to their power as mothers over their children within the domestic domain. She describes this as the key to explaining women's violence towards their children and, quoting Dally, says: 'Today's mother probably has total power over her child, and over no one and nothing else. She is exposed to the full impact of her personality' (p. 165).

Children therefore become the nearest target for the outlet of the frustrations, anger and guilt of their mothers. It is not necessarily easy for health visitors and other nurses to, on the one hand, retain an understanding of the pressures which lead mothers to exercise their power over children, and on the other hand recognise and assert children's rights to freedom from violence and humiliation. Can we continue to sacrifice children? Both children and parents need help in learning how to safely experience and cope with anger.

In the first years of children's lives, health visitors and community nurses are in a unique position to help parents examine their own needs, while also acknowledging the child's point of view as an individual with separate individual needs. Parents are often asking for more effective ways of managing their children's behaviour. The best opportunities lie with the new young family, before punishments are firmly established as a method of helping children learn how to behave, and before mother has learned the automatic smack response, which becomes as easy as changing gear in the car (Pound, 1991). This is not an easy task when the pressure from the rest of society constantly reaffirms the notion that without a firm hand parental control will be lost. Many mothers will learn to use smacking from their own mothers and other close contacts who can be more influential than the health visitor and community nurse. A legal ban would demonstrate that society forbade all degrees of physical punishment, no matter how small as a matter of principle. Health visitors and other nurses could then be seen as working with parents rather than against them and their personal 'right' to smack (Cook et al., 1991). It is important to challenge clearly the use of physical punishments as a method of teaching children right from wrong, otherwise it remains an option to be used. However, open disapproval of little smacks is probably counter-productive. To respond to parental requests for help in managing specific situations is likely to be more effective than talking about principles with individuals.

Parents living in conditions of material deprivation, with low income, difficult, overcrowded housing, and stressful relationships, may of course find it more difficult to learn these skills because life itself is more difficult for them. It is not impossible or too much to ask of these parents, but they will need much more support to achieve results. Positive parenting (Cook et al., 1991) can be approached from a self-interest point of view by showing parents they will experience fewer stressful scenes, more agreeable children, and warmer relationships with a greater sense of achievement. Working sympathetically with parents as issues arise will be perceived by them as practical help. Similarly, parents need help in recognising age-appropriate behaviour for each stage of child development and what they can realistically expect.

Group work with parents, most likely mothers' groups, provides opportunities for discussion about the principles of children's rights and for exploration of childhood learning processes and child development. They can also provide for women's solidarity, so that women can share experiences and support each other in understanding the pressures of mothering.

In the current political climate surrounding children and their rights, when aims are to raise public awareness and encourage legal reforms, health visitors and community nurses also need to grasp the nettle and reach the wider public through the media, public meetings and street stalls.

Considering what to teach

Large amounts of adult behaviour have a basis of learning in childhood. Learning is a gradual process which continues throughout life and is constantly modified and reviewed according to changing experiences. Children are not born with automatic knowledge of the difference between right and wrong, just as they are not born pre-programmed to be selfish, and it is generally agreed that environment and experiences of daily living play an important part in social development. It is also agreed that people have a need for approval, affection and to be valued as individuals in order to foster self-esteem.

Positive discipline is training which will eventually produce self-control and does not involve punishment. Control imposed through the fear of being caught is not true self-control. Equally, if no boundaries are put on behaviour, children lack the opportunity to learn respect for others. Children learn how to live and behave in society in the same way that they learn everything else, with information and guidelines, by trial and error, practice and, importantly, with reinforcements for getting it right. It is unrealistic to expect children to remember after hearing something just once and thereafter be blindly obedient. (If children were so capable, they would be potty trained and learn to read quicker than they do!) Children are most likely to behave well if they are given the information in advance and then receive acknowledgement. The command 'don't touch that' will be more effective if accompanied by an explanation followed by an acknowledgement that the child did well not to touch. Children will make mistakes, but usually punishments of any sort should be a last option, because people learn more reliable lessons from positive reinforcements. Atkinson et al. (1990) state that for punishments to work they must be immediate, as early as possible in the behaviour, and mild, with the least amount of emotion; the punishment must also provide a recognisable alternative which is then reinforced. Until children are old enough to understand explanations they will also need to be kept safe and diverted from danger. Safety equipment such as fire-guards, stair gates and children's reins help avoid conflicts. Evasive action in the interest of safety does not need to contain an element of punishment. Unfortunately, if parents find that a smack does stop a behaviour, they are more likely to use it again. This is why they need help to find more effective methods of steering, motivating and retraining. Unrealistic expectations of young children's capabilities are more likely to arise from ignorance than malice. Parents may need help to understand how much children are capable of learning at different ages.

The example set from the memory of our own childhood is extremely persuasive. It is difficult to question what your parents did to you, or believe that their punishments were not necessary when as a young child you thought them infallible. Young children automatically hold their parents in high regard simply because they are the closest and most influential model there is to copy.

Repeatedly, adults say of punishments administered to them by their parents 'it never did me any harm', and 'I deserved what I got'. This illustrates the faith children have in adults. The overall conclusion of a large study of young people receiving help from a social service department was that 'even recipients of extremely punitive discipline fail to recognise the inappropriateness of specific acts of discipline . . . while they describe the identical discipline of others as abusive' (Berger et al., 1988).

At stake here is the need to be valued by others whom you respect and upon whom you are dependent. But children continue to be treated as possessions of their parents, thus relegating them to a second-class status and denying them equal respect. As yet one more illustration, Yule's research, conducted through observing people in public places, found that although adults are usually courteous to other adults there is widespread rudeness towards children (1985).

The stereotype of parents barely surviving their less-than-delightful children with an air of martyrdom is reinforced by models on television and by cartoonists like Posy Simmonds. Violence towards others as a way of problem-solving continues to have a firm hold in escapist television and films. Even presenters of children's BBC freely clout 'Edd the duck' about the head. A hierarchy of authority still exists in this country, and children are at the bottom. I believe that children have a basic need to be able to learn in a warm, encouraging environment with clear guidelines and positive reinforcements which foster self-esteem. Children should have, as of right, equal protection under the law from humiliating and degrading experiences and all forms of violence, even from their parents. This requires a change in the status of children so that they receive equal respect as individuals.

References

Atkinson, R. et al. (1990) *Introduction to Psychology*. Florida: Harcourt Brace Jovanovich.

Bandura, A. (1973) *Aggression: A Social Learning Analysis*. Englewood Cliffs, NJ: Prentice Hall.

Bandura, A. (1977) *Social Learning Theory*. Englewood Cliffs, NJ: Prentice Hall.

Bandura, A., Ross, D. and Ross, S. (1973) The transmission of aggression through imitation of aggressive models. In E. Aronson, *Readings about the Social Animal*. San Francisco: Freeman.

Baumrind, D. and Black, A. (1967) Socialization practices associates with dimensions of competence in preschool boys and girls. *Child Development*, 38, pp. 291–327.

Berger, A. et al. (1988) The self report of punitive childhood experiences of young adults and adolescents. *Child Abuse and Neglect*, 12 (2) pp. 251–62.

Calam, R. and Franchi, C. (1987) *Child Abuse and its Consequences*. Cambridge: Cambridge University Press.

Cook, A., James, J. and Leach, P. (1991) *Positively No Smacking*. London: Health Visitors Association.

Coopersmith, S. (1967) *The Antecedents of Self Esteem*. San Francisco: Freeman.

Creighton, S. J. (1984) *Trends in Child Abuse 1977–82: The Fourth Report on the Children placed on the NSPCC Special Unit Registers*. London: National Society for the Prevention of Cruelty to Children.

Dally, Ann quoted in C. Webb (1986) Op Cit.

POCH (End Physical Punishment of Children) (1990) *Child Abuse and Physical Punishment: Report of UK Social Services and Social Work Departments on Policies and Practice Regarding Physical Punishment and Perceptions of its Relationship to Child Abuse*. London: APPROACH.

Eron, L. (1987) The development of aggressive behaviour from the perspective of a developing behaviourism. In R. Atkinson et al., *Introduction to Psychology*. Florida: Harcourt Brace Jovanovich.

Gallup Poll (1989) *Attitudes Towards Punishing Children*. Commissioned by EPOCH (End Physical Punishment of Children).

Jones, D., Pickett, J., Oates, M. and Barbor, P. (1987) *Understanding Child Abuse*. 2nd edn. London: Macmillan.

Miller, A. (1987) *For Your own Good: The Roots of Violence in Child Rearing*. London: Virago.

Newell, P. (1989) *Children Are People Too: The Case Against Physical Punishment*. London: Bedford Square.

Newell, P. (1991) *Convention and Children's Rights in the UK*. London: National Children's Bureau.

Newson, J. and Newson, E. (1989) *The Extent of Physical Punishment in the UK*. London: APPROACH.

Ong, B. N. (1986) Are abusing women abused women? In C. Webb (ed.), *Feminist Practice in Women's Health Care*. Chichester: Wiley & Sons.

Orr, J. (1986) Feminism and health visiting. In C. Webb (ed.), *Feminist Practice in Women's Health Care*. Chichester: Wiley & Sons.

Peters, R. S. (1981) *Moral Development and Moral Education*. London: Allen and Unwin.

Pound, R. (1991) Positively no smacking. *Health Visitor*, 64, 9, pp. 289–91.

Rogers, C. and Stevens, B. (1967) *Person to Person: The Problem of Being Human*. New York: Pocket Books.

Wolfe, D. (1987 and 1989) *Implications for Child Development and Psychopathology*. Newbury Park, Ca: Sage.

Yule, V. (1985) Why are parents tough on children? *New Society*, 73, 1187.

4 Partnership and professional power

Carole Peall

> A good pass? Did he say a good pass? I could have had a better
> result blindfolded.

A typical Saturday afternoon's entertainment for me is listening to my
son arguing with the professional commentator on television about
the game of, you guessed, football! Having suffered many such
afternoons, I realise I have produced unwittingly I might add, a child
for whom a constant barrage of arguments with a professional expert
is a prime source of enjoyment. I confess that I too have such (one-
sided) arguments, being particularly susceptible when behind the
wheel of my car. There are many such situations in which we all claim
to have superior knowledge over others in our everyday lives: the 'we
know best' syndrome. As professionals we no doubt lay claim to
possession of professional expertise and knowledge too. The concept
and practice of working in a partnership with our clients, very much
in vogue at the moment, has to some extent thrown into sharp relief
our claims regarding superior knowledge and hence power over our
clients. This chapter will explore some of the contradictions inherent
in commonly held notions of professional expertise and lay knowledge
with reference to child protection issues, and focus upon the concept
of professional/client partnership as a means of exemplifying these.

A short history of the partnership principle in community nursing

Many developments have contributed towards adoption of the concept of partnership with clients in the sphere of community nursing (as well as in other professional spheres). Perhaps a first step along this pathway of putting the principle of partnership into practice began with the introduction of Walter Barker's Child Development Programme in the 1980s. This programme was based upon the notion that health visitors could, and should, work alongside parents of young children, each acknowledging the other's expertise, sharing information and insights and pooling their resources in the best interests of the child. The programme has proved to be a resounding success with both parents and health visitors alike and has illustrated that it is possible for two sometimes different perspectives to co-exist in mutual harmony and benefit.

Another impetus to the partnership principle came through the creation of the idea and format for parent-held child health records from a joint inter-professional working party convened by the British Paediatric Association (1990). These records were originally piloted in the Oxfordshire Health Authority, and thorough evaluation of the scheme again highlighted the benefits of sharing the information held on health records and the value of partnership between professionals and clients (Saffin, 1986; McFarlane and Saffin, 1990a, 1990b). Many health authorities throughout the UK have now implemented parent-held child health records, or are moving towards their implementation, and the Health Visitors Association and the Royal College of Nursing, the professional organisations for health visitors and community nurses, formally support and encourage this move (Health Visitors Association, 1991a).

Recent changes in legislation have given further momentum to the principle of partnership between professional and client. The Access to Health Records Act, implemented in November 1991, gives patients and clients access to information held on them on all manual health records *by right* (except in very rare circumstances). The Children Act 1989 also expressly encourages the principles and practice of partnership between parents, children and the professional workers with whom they are in contact. Courts and professionals must now listen to, consult with, and take into account the views of both children and their parents at all stages of child protection proceedings, including when children are looked after in long-term local authority care placements (Health Visitors Association, 1991b; Hayes and Naish, 1992). Recent national guidance on child protection work, *Working Together*, also emphasises the partnership principle,

and indeed extends and further builds upon the legislative framework, stating, for example, that parents should normally be invited to
attend child protection case conferences: 'While there may be
exceptional occasions when it will not be right to invite one or other
parent to attend a case conference in whole or in part, exclusion
should be kept to a minimum and needs to be especially justified'
(Department of Health, 1991, p. 43).

Last, but not least, clients themselves and the general public at
large have increasingly demanded an equal partnership with the
professionals they meet. They want the opportunity to share information fully, select the options they feel most appropriate to them, and
participate in any decisions made about their care. Perhaps one of the
most developed and best examples of this consumer movement is that
surrounding women's right to participate in decisions made about
their health care whilst they are pregnant, a movement often loosely
associated with the National Childbirth Trust. Obstetricians and
other doctors are increasingly now no longer in the position of being
able to dictate to women where or how they will give birth. There is
every sign that such consumer demands will spread to children as a
consumer group too, with the recent establishment of the Children's
Rights Development Unit in London (see chapter 3 for further
discussion of children's rights).

So the partnership principle seems here to stay. But what does this
mean for community nurses and health visitors working in the child
protection area? And, importantly, will such partnerships bring about
a confrontation or a harmony between the different views and
knowledge of nurses, health visitors and parents in the sensitive and
emotion-ridden areas of child abuse? And are these views and
knowledge so different anyway? Let us look at the issue of parental
participation in child protection case conferences to explore these
questions further.

Parental participation at child protection case conferences

Most local authorities now routinely invite parents to attend child
protection case conferences. Prior to this, most had had some form of
compromise, parents being invited to input into the case conference
not in person but via a third party, usually their social worker. Full or
part participation by parents at case conferences has caused some
gasps of astonishment and much anxiety in community nursing (and
no doubt other professional disciplines too). They have felt that a
previous professional-only domain was threatened by the, in some
cases, enforced invitation of parents to join them. Professionals voiced

their reluctance to encourage this participation in terms of the 'best interests of the child', and envisaged problems which centred around the confidentiality of information and inability to fully share their perceptions, and the perceived threat of violence to themselves or others. All are genuine concerns.

Confidentiality and sharing information

If we look at the perceived problem of confidentiality, perhaps we would be justified in looking first at the question of sharing information with other agencies. Many battles have been fought in the past between different agencies over who owns information on clients. This conflict has now extended to the parents instead. The answer to the question 'Do professionals have exclusive rights to knowledge of the child?' must surely be 'no', since if we as professionals do not share our general knowledge of the child with the carers concerned, we are unable to check out the accuracy of our beliefs. Research carried out in Gloucestershire into views of professionals, following 65 child protection case conferences which the parents also attended, suggested that professionals found the experience largely positive with few negative connotations (Burns, 1991). However, community nurses, health visitors and other professionals, who have not yet experienced full parental participation at case conferences, often imagine the worst possible scenario, which would perhaps be that the parents found the information being offered to be so incorrect that they sued the individual concerned for libel. This is an extreme example, but one which professionals do express concern about: if information were imparted which was totally unfounded and inaccurate, the parents would have every right to challenge the professional.

A milder, and perhaps more likely scenario, is that parents challenge the foundations of the professionals' view, for example, challenging the accuracy of observations and/or re-interpretating the meaning of events such as lack of obvious physical affection between parent and child. And it is actually very important to allow this to happen. Indeed, it should be positively encouraged! This is partly because parents may well be right and able to demonstrate the validity of their point of view, particularly given the fact that professionals only obtain a 'snapshot' picture of the family lives of others and are therefore not necessarily able to construct a comprehensive and whole picture of the child and the parent–child relationship in the same way that parents are able to. It is also because, whether the parents' point of view is judged to be valid or not, expression of their point of view allows professionals to gain understanding of where they are coming from in terms of their perspectives, beliefs, and values on parenting, childhood, and so on. And this surely gives the professionals concerned an opportunity and a starting point for developing further supportive work, which in turn is one of the central aims of a case conference. Also, and of equal importance, parents are allowed to see where *you* are coming from as a professional and what your expectations and standards are in relation to parenting skills.

Violence

The threat of violence to professional workers is another concern voiced in relation to parental participation at child protection case conferences. There is certainly some foundation for these concerns. Thea Brown's research in 1987 in the area of physical child abuse revealed that violence towards the child was often not an isolated incident and usually indicated other acts of violence within the family setting (1991). Indeed, there is a wealth of evidence which suggests that violence manifested by adults is often linked to child abuse both in terms of adults' own experiences of child abuse (Gelles and Podrick Connell, 1990; Berger et al., 1988) and their further perpetration of abuse and violence towards their own children (Strauss et al., 1980). The fear of violence expressed by professionals is thus a very real one. However, parents are unlikely to be violent towards an individual professional within the context of a case conference at which other professionals are also present, or at least any such violence manifested could be contained. The necessity for violence is, anyway, considerably defused through communication, in which all parties concerned can express their observations, perspectives, feelings and views, and gain understanding of each other's position. Research clearly indicates that the risk of aggressive behaviour is considerably reduced when precipitated by other means of more appropriate and adequate communication (Leiba, 1987; Smith, 1988).

Participation and knowledge

What actually is participation, and what does it mean in the context of parental participation at child protection case conferences? A definitive answer appears to elude us. As research in the London Borough of Hackney (Hackney Social Services, 1990), which examined parental participation at case conferences, put it:

> Unlike concepts such as 'power' or 'democracy', 'participation' has escaped almost any semantic, philosophical, sociological or psychological analysis. The word appears in many publications yet it is, often, used interchangeably with 'involvement' and 'attendance'. But does a participant at a case conference mean something different by merely being present? (p. 11)

The concept of participation in this context is thus entwined with that of knowledge, more specifically respect for, and consideration of, the knowledge parents bring with them to case conferences.

Knowledge, in this context, includes more than just information; it also involves knowing about specific group behaviours, and mores, rites and rituals of case conferences. Failure to achieve this state will leave parents feeling excluded and they will not experience partnership. (p. 11)

Parents will also need to feel mutuality with the professionals present and believe that they are being treated as fellow citizens by them. Whatever the nature of the alleged or actual abuse, the parents should not experience being 'looked down on', marginalised or oppressed by the professionals. If this occurs they will experience feelings of isolation, exclusion and non-partnership.

Thus, professionals need to *value* the 'lay' knowledge parents have in respect of their children if they are ever to achieve 'partnership' with them in any meaningful sense. This in turn has consequences for the traditional hierarchy and balance of power between professionals and clients, i.e. professional expertise as superior to lay knowledge, and puts clients much more on the same footing as professionals. Some might perceive this as a direct attack on their professional status and authority. But if we stop to consider where our knowledge is derived from, especially in the field of child care, we will ascertain that much comes from our own experience of parenting and/or childhood, much of the remainder stemming from the collective experiences of parents (particularly mothers) and children themselves, whether gleaned and distilled from a textbook, lecture or professional contact. It seems to me to be both ludicrous and artificial to imagine we acquire professional knowledge in any other way, albeit a version of professional knowledge which is often given the gloss and aura of scientism in order to elevate its status and separate it from the rank of everyday experience.

If, as community nurses and health visitors, we are to truly provide care in a holistic sense, we must be prepared to acknowledge, recognise and indeed encourage the combination of professional and lay knowledge in order to create an environment in which both professionals and clients, be they adults or children, can reach their potential. The majority of parents want the best for their children, even parents who have abused their children. Surely we share that aim?

References

Berger, A. et al. (1988) The self report of punitive childhood experiences of young adults and adolescents. *Child Abuse and Neglect, 12 (2) pp. 251–62.*

British Paediatric Association (1990) *Report of the Joint Working Party on professional and Parent-Held Records used in Child Health Surveillance*. London: British Paediatric Association.

Brown, T. (1991) Unpublished paper, British Association of the Study and Prevention Child Abuse and Neglect (BASPCAN) Conference, Leicester.

Burns, L. (1991) *Partnership with Families*. Gloucester: Gloucestershire County Council Social Services.

Department of Health (1991) *Working Together under The Children Act 1989*. London: HMSO.

Gelles, R. and Podrick Connell, C. (1990) *Intimate Violence in Families*. 2nd edn, Newberry Park: Sage.

Hackney Social Services (1990) *Parental Participation in Child Protection Conferences*. Norwich: University of East Anglia.

Hayes, E. and Naish, J. (1992) *Keeping Children Safe*. London: Health Visitors Association/National Society for the Prevention of Cruelty to Children.

Health Visitors Association (1991a) *In Their Own Hands*. London: Health Visitors Association.

Health Visitors Association (1991b) *The Children Act 1989: Guidance on Professional Practice*. London: Health Visitors Association.

Leiba, P. (1987) Violence: the community nurses dilemma. *Health Visitor*, 60, November, pp. 361–2.

McFarlane, A. and Saffin, K. (1990a) Do general practitioners and health visitors like parent-held child health records? *British Journal of General Practice*, 40, pp. 106–8.

McFarlane, A. and Saffin, K. (1990b) How well are parent-held records kept and completed? *British Journal of General Practice*, 41, pp. 249–51.

Saffin, K. (1986) Parents as partners. *Community Outlook*, February, pp. 21–22.

Smith, S. (1988) Take care, be aware. *Community Outlook*, March.

Strauss, M.A., Gelles, R. and Steinmetz, S. S. (1980) *Behind Closed Doors: Violence in the American Family*. New York: Anchor/Doubleday.

5   Supervision versus control: can managers provide both managerial and professional supervision?

Jane Parkinson

The conflicting needs and differing responsibilities of community nursing staff and their managers have not, to date, been sufficiently addressed in national guidelines. As the concept and practice of general management becomes increasingly established, will it be possible, feasible or even desirable to continue to combine professional and managerial supervision? This chapter considers the differences between managerial and professional supervision, and includes research evidence from a project designed to investigate this issue in relation to child protection work (Taket et al., 1990).

The particular questions which will be discussed here are:

- can line managers, by the very nature of their task, fulfil the supervision needs of community nursing staff working with abusing families?
- can a line manager provide a safe environment for a community nurse in which to explore her feelings around abuse? Is this necessary in this area of work?
- can the line manager enable community nurses to work in the most flexible and effective way whilst simultaneously being

responsible for appraising staff performance and measuring the quality and effectiveness of the service provided? Is this asking too much of the manager and community nurse alike?

These are questions I considered whilst working as a nurse specialist in child protection in Tower Hamlets. It came to my attention that community nurse managers were supervising child protection casework for about 28 staff each, and overall there were around 80 children on the child protection register, with another 240 families in which there was concern regarding the future possibility of abuse. At this time, North East Thames Regional Health Authority, in which my district was located, issued a policy statement on child protection (1988). This included a section for nurse managers which stated their role as encompassing regular review and monitoring of all case records, case discussion, and attendance at all case conferences attended by nurses.

The impossibility of carrying out this policy without excessive management workload and/or an almost complete exclusion of other management functions precipitated a management crisis in Tower Hamlets Health Authority. The policy statement also seemed to be one step further towards restricting and controlling community nurses, rather than enabling, empowering and supporting them to take professional responsibility for their own work. However, this management crisis created an opportunity for research and new thinking on what supervision actually consisted of for nursing practice in the area of child protection work and also whom it benefited.

Meanings and definitions of supervisions

What is supervision? Clearly, it seemed necessary to separate out management and fieldworker requirements in supervision.

The benefits of supervision for an individual worker are summed up in the report on the death of Kimberley Carlile: 'However experienced a worker it is possible to get stuck, confused, frightened or bored. The task of supervision is to be watchful for these signs.' (London Borough of Greenwich and Greenwich Health Authority, 1987, p. 193).

Interestingly, the report divides the supervision of social work staff into twin components: managerial supervision and professional supervision. Managerial supervision is defined in the report as monitoring policies, resources, and service provision; and professional supervision as ensuring field staff respond to individual cases appropriately, take into account the specific context and needs of the child and family, yet retain their objectivity. These same two components of supervision could be applied to the work of community nurses in child protection.

On this basis, the content and requirements of managerial supervision might include:

1 monitoring the levels of known child abuse;
2 ensuring effective and appropriate local procedures and policies in child protection work are in place in order to provide a safe framework for practice;
3 identifying the education and training needs of staff and facilitating means of meeting these;
4 measuring the quality and effectiveness of service provision;
5 appraising the performance of individual workers in child protection work, in part through observation and discussion of case records;
6 assessing the resources staff need in order to carry out their work;
7 ensuring staff are provided with and have access to professional supervision.

The above list of requirements is relatively uncontroversial. However, it does not necessarily take into account the feelings and emotions engendered within individual professionals when dealing with the abuse of children — feelings and experiences which are essential to acknowledge and explore within a safe environment in order that the professional may retain objectivity in her assessment of the child's family situation and offer the most appropriate form of support and advice. This is a core element of professional supervision which the Kimberley Carlile report had in mind:

> Supervision enables practitioners to know themselves. We all have some areas of our work we find more difficult than others; we all have weaknesses as well as strengths. (London Borough of Greenwich and Greenwich Health Authority, 1987, p. 192)

Hawkins and Shohat similarly state that workers who are engaged in intimate and therepeutic work with clients are:

> Necessarily allowing themselves to be affected by the distress, pain and fragmentation of the client and need time to become aware of how this has affected them and to deal with any reactions . . . Not attending to these emotions soon leads to less than effective workers, who become either over-identified with their clients or defended against being further affected by them. This in time leads to stress and what is commonly called burn out. (1989, p. 42)

Thus, professional workers with abusing families are in danger of losing their objectivity and/or closing off channels of communication with families, so inhibiting the development of appropriate means of support. The aim of professional supervision might therefore revolve around the facilitation and enablement of professionals to discuss their feelings and emotions *in relation to* their professional practice, professional responsibilities and work objectives for individual children/families.

We can therefore see that there are clearly two components involved within staff supervision in the protection of children. However, the professional component of supervision as outlined above has largely been ignored within the arena of nursing and health visitor practice. Indeed, the Department of Health stated in its guidance to senior nurses on child protection work that supervision meant:

> To assess the workload of practitioners, both individually and as a group; to measure the quality and effectiveness of their work, to set and monitor standards of practice, and to give professional advice and monitor training. (1988, p. 33)

This statement appears to address only the needs of management by promoting the monitoring of staff performance without acknowledging, or indeed allowing for, the fact that community nurses are human beings dealing with vulnerable children and families, *all* of whom need safe support in order to effect change. The separation of supervision functions into the two elements of professional and managerial supervision may rectify the latter situation. But can one person perform both functions appropriately? And more particularliy, can a nurse manager, given the structural context of her relationship to her nursing staff, effectively provide a professional supervision service? This is something we set out to discover in Tower Hamlets Health Authority.

The Tower Hamlets Health Authority project on child protection supervision

As previously stated, the North East Thames Regional Health Authority policy paper highlighted a management crisis for the supervision of field staff in their child protection work. The nurse managers could not undertake the supervision functions outlined in this document due to the sheer volume of work it would entail. And they were certainly not in a position to extend their role and work further into professional supervision. It was decided to call upon community nurses who were experienced in child protection work to undertake some of these functions and a six-month pilot project was agreed. A philosophy behind this project was that such nurses were ideally placed to offer their peers professional supervision. The overall objectives of this project were therefore to: relieve the management situation regarding supervision of child protection work; review and evaluate the system of child protection overall by looking at different ways of working and aiming to empower staff and enable them to recognise and take responsibility for themselves in this area of work.

Through the creation of specific employment posts for supervision of nurses in child protection work by their experienced peers, posts known as child protection advisers (CPA), it was hoped that nurse managers would be freed to examine their role in supervision as nurse managers and to develop areas such as staff appraisal systems. It was hoped also that community nurses would, as a consequence, be better supported in their work.

The aims of the project were therefore to:

- offer increased professional advice and support to field staff and managers in the area of child protection;
- reduce field staff and management stress in the child protection component of their work;
- provide an increased emphasis on self-referral by staff for support, and provide on-going support in a flexible way;
- value and empower staff and recognise the work undertaken by them.

The project was designed to be evaluated by an outside researcher in order to determine any change in nursing and staff attitudes, including their perceptions of the type of support and advice offered.

The child protection advisers

Following much debate, it was decided that health visitors should have access to a CPA with a health visitor background, and that school nurses should have access to a CPA with a school nursing background. It was also decided that CPAs should work in their capacity as advisers for half their working time, maintaining clinical 'hands-on' work with clients for the rest of their working time. Both these decisions were taken in order that CPAs kept up-to-date in knowledge and skills relating to their own disciplinary area of practice, maintained realistic expectations of their peers' practice, and also retained credibility with their own peer group. CPAs were formally interviewed for appointment to their post. They had to demonstrate in-depth knowledge of child protection policy and practice issues, in addition to well-developed skills of communication (especially ability to listen), problem solving, organisation and team building, in order to achieve appointment. Each CPA was to support the work of ten of her peers in the field.

A training programme for the newly appointed CPA was then constructed. The training programme was centrally based upon the Open University Child Abuse and Neglect course (1990), which is specifically designed to develop an understanding of child abuse with regard to personal feelings, experiences and values in relation to personal and professional judgements and actions. Other aspects of the CPA training centred around:

- developing communication skills
- professional responsibility and accountability, including that associated with poor standards of practice
- group work and individual casework
- legislative frameworks, including the court setting
- record keeping and report writing
- participating in case conferences
- negotiating contracts with families and setting objectives for practice
- means and methods of self-support

Professional accountability

A key element of the project was the underlying principle of professional accountability. Health visitors and community nurses needed to be made aware that *they* were responsible for their individual practice with families, including all actions they took (or did not take). It was important to emphasise to them that the creation of CPA posts in no way exonerated their responsibilities in respect of their own professional accountability for practice (UK Central Council for Nurses, Midwives and Health Visitors, 1989).

However, the CPAs also had responsibilities in respect of their professional accountability with regard to the observation, supervision, advice and support they offered to their peers. They needed to first demonstrate to their peers that they had adopted safe and high standards of practice. As Jones et al. have put it in relation to the supervisor as a role model: '. . . the supervisor should demonstrate in the organisation of *his* work how staff should relate to the families *they* supervise' (1987, p. 241; my italics).

The question that next arose was what happens in the event of unsafe or poor practice being identified. Issues highlighted that might arise were:

- a community nurse failing to identify any causes for concern in families within her caseload
- inadequate documentation, including not preparing reports for case conferences
- no proof of pro-active practice service offered to clients, i.e. not making contracts with clients or setting joint objectives
- not following procedures and working within national and local guidelines for good practice
- not making comprehensive or adequate assessments of the family.

Protocols were agreed whereby the concerns about individual nursing practice held by CPAs would be assessed as to whether this reflected a training need, for example not understanding procedures, and whether it was within agreed safety margins. If a situation became chronic, or practice was considered unsafe, the CPA would initiate a joint meeting with the nurse specialist for child protection and the member of staff concerned.

The nurse specialist would make a decision on how to then proceed, thus avoiding confusion with respect to the responsibilities of managerial supervision and professional supervision.

Evaluation of the project

A questionnaire was developed to be completed by all nurse managers and all community nursing and health visiting staff. The management questionnaire focused upon the amount and type of work spent on child protection, whilst the questionnaire to staff focused upon how the child protection advisers functioned as a staff resource. The questionnaire thus covered areas such as freedom to discuss as many cases as they wished, levels of stress and confidence experienced, and the way they were currently working with families. Both questionnaires were completed anonymously prior to the project commencing, and at the end of the six-month period.

The independent researcher interviewed a sample of field staff, nurse managers and the CPAs in depth in the last month of the project. In addition, Table 5.1 from manager questionnaires illustrates the workload indicators for nurse managers. The managers retained responsibility for a quarter of their staff in terms of child protection supervision work. Their perceived workload was reduced by 50 per cent, except in the number of hours spent on other related child protection issues, which is to be expected as general issues such as paediatric liaison, social service meetings and policy meetings are still the responsibility of nurse managers.

Table 5.1 Child protection workload indicators for managers, in two four week periods before and during the CPA project, totals for all managers shown

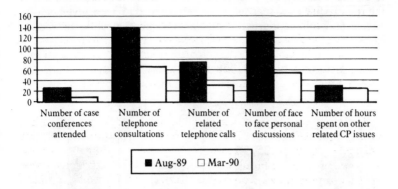

Source: Taket, A. et al. (1990)

Table 5.2, constructed from data available from the questionnaire to field staff, illustrates the percentage of staff able to discuss as many cases as they liked. Before the project started, 40 per cent of staff felt they were unable to discuss as many child protection cases as they would have liked. Six months later, only 15 per cent of staff felt unable to discuss as many cases as they would have liked. This included nursing and health visitor staff still supervised solely by their nurse managers without access to a CPA.

Table 5.2 Percentage of staff who were able to discuss as many cases as they liked in the preceding six months

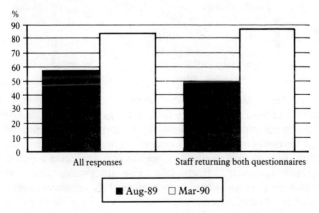

Source: Taket, A. et al. (1990)

Table 5.3, again from data obtained from the questionnaire to field staff, shows the changes in positive outcomes in response to a request to discuss a family. As is seen, six months into the project more staff felt their request was met helpfully, felt listened to, were given helpful advice and felt supported in the management of child protection cases.

Table 5.3   Changes in positive outcomes in response to request to discuss a family

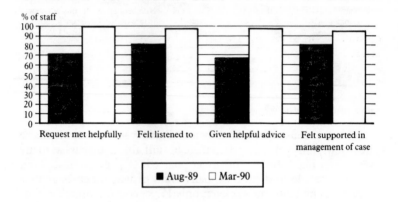

Source: Taket, A. et al. (1990)

The following further findings are taken from in-depth interviews carried out with health authority staff. The sample was drawn in such a way as to ensure it included:

- nursing staff allocated to a CPA, and nursing staff allocated to a nurse manager for provision of child protection advice;
- both school nurses and health visitors;
- nursing staff from all areas of the district;
- nursing staff with variable amounts of experience in both child protection work and time spent employed within the district.

Staff who were interviewed were assured that anything they said would be treated in confidence and that no individuals would be identified in the report. The emphasis throughout interviews was on seeking the views of all staff on how the scheme had functioned, its impact on them as professionals, as well as exploration of views about reasons for any such effects felt. The interviews provided an opportunity to explore in more depth some of the areas covered in the written questionnaire.

The first area explored in detail was staff's experience of child protection work and advice on it over the six-month experimental period of the CPA project.

Responses were analyzed in relation to any perceived differences in experience between nursing staff allocated to a CPA separate from their manager and nursing staff who had received advice on child protection directly from line managers. Those staff who had been allocated a CPA separate from their manager were, without exception, positive about their overall experience of the scheme. All found it beneficial in some ways. This applied *equally* to those staff who reported experiencing some negative or potentially negative expectations about the scheme before it was implemented as well as those who reported only positive expectations of the scheme before its start. All of those reporting negative or potentially negative expectations of the scheme went on to say they had not been borne out in practice. Key aspects that were mentioned *repeatedly* as positive were the CPA's easy accessibility and the ease of availability of informal advice and support. The separation of the CPA role from the post of nurse manager was perceived as particularly beneficial in the above because staff felt more able to seek help from someone who was not also their manager and therefore not responsible for the individual performance appraisal. The following typical comments illustrate this:

> It's particularly helpful that . . . she's not a manager, I don't feel her breathing down my neck. I can be honest with her about my shortcomings, not feel threatened . . . able to be more honest with her, and therefore get more help.

> . . . She's not the person appraising you, that's important . . . more openness is possible with a CPA. (Taket et al., 1990, p. 34)

The CPAs were seen as supportive by staff, providing them with opportunities to consider options and courses of action and to check out their views and perceptions, whilst still retaining overall control and responsibility for their own work. Connected to the notion of receiving support in their work whilst remaining in control of it, staff valued the *manner* in which CPAs offered advice and support characterising this with terms such as 'not patronising', 'non-judgemental', 'non-prescriptive', 'non-directive'. When the issue of responsibility for child protection work was talked about, *all* of the nursing staff with the CPA identified the responsibility for ensuring that child protection work is carried out for their clients as their *own*. Some staff explicitly contrasted this with the situation before the project, commenting that they felt managers took on, or took over, responsibility for child protection work once they had been brought into contact with it.

Another important element which emerged in the staff's views of the function of their CPA was *their* confidence in the knowledge and experience of the CPAs. This was linked by many of the staff to the CPAs being drawn from the same professional background as themselves, so that the CPA had direct experience of the role and remit of the member of staff concerned and knew the context in which they worked. These points were also emphasised when staff talked about how they would like to see child protection advice provided in the future.

The ready availability of a trusted person who could be relied upon to advise and support staff was identified by many of those interviewed as being instrumental in ensuring safe practice in child protection. And in this connection, staff thought their readiness to utilise CPA services was particularly important. Staff also commented on the benefit of the CPAs retaining a clinical caseload as they felt it extremely relevant that CPAs had kept in touch with fieldwork. One disadvantage of this was that staff sometimes felt reluctant to disturb a CPA if they knew she was working with her own client caseload.

Some particular areas of practice that were described as helpful, mentioned several times by different staff, were:

- help with planning and preparing for case conferences (an area identified by several staff as being particularly difficult and stressful);
- support in participating at case conferences;
- confirmation and reassurances about action planned;
- supportive work with families in which there were causes for concern but not proven child abuse (another area identified by several staff as being particularly difficult and stressful);
- clarification of views, perceptions and opinions;
- exploration of options for future action and practice;
- facilitation of change to work with families in different ways (a particular benefit perceived by staff was that they felt able to undertake more pro-active, rather than mere reactive, work).

Eleven out of thirteen staff interviewed who had been allocated to a CPA had also experienced contact with them in groups as well as on an individual basis. Activities carried out within groups varied but included discussion of particular topics, for example: working openly with families; discussion of cases — hypothetical or real; simulated exercises and role-play to facilitate sharing experiences and comparing views. Staff viewed these groups as having two different functions: firstly, that of continuing training and education, including opportunities for practice development; and secondly, that of providing support and reducing feelings of isolation in relation to child protection work. The group work component was a *highly* valued part of the overall scheme, for both these two perceived functions.

Staff were also asked about their feelings towards child protection work and whether these had changed over the past six months. Eleven out of thirteen staff reported positive changes, typically a reduction in stress and anxiety levels and an improvement in confidence; many of these staff commented that they felt more supported in their work and more relaxed and able to deal with it.

Staff allocated solely to a nurse manager for child protection supervision reported a much lower level of contact over the six-month period than the staff allocated to a CPA. This difference did not seem to be related to the level or intensity of child protection work associated with a current caseload, since the range of variation in this was very similar to that found with staff allocated to a CPA. There was a much lower incidence of both group work and reviews of casework with individual families who gave cause for professional concern. Staff also mentioned difficulties or frustrations on occasions when they tried to make contact with their manager for child protection advice and support.

Nurse managers reported that they had not been able to devote as much time to their child protection work as they would have liked owing to competing demands which arose from other parts of their managerial roles. The managers reported no difficulties in separating their managerial role from the advice and support role for those members of staff for whom they retained both functions, but commented in several places that they thought staff may have found difficulties in fully utilising the advice and support role owing to the combination of roles. The existence of a separate person giving child protection advice to staff meant considerable changes for all managers in their workloads. Comments made by the managers on the effects of this included:

enabled me to become more of a manager

If we'd not lost the child protection work, I would have to have said I can't do this job any more.

Before the scheme I was so wound up about child protection it dominated my working life and spilled over into my personal life; giving it up has enabled me to talk to staff about other things. (Taket et al., 1990, p. 42)

The managers were very positive about the provision of advice and support to staff outside line management. They felt this was very beneficial for their staff, and improved the availability and accessibility of advice and support. Positive comments received by managers on the development of child protection work by their staff included:

much more field worker lead and owned

staff and clients enabled to work in a contractual way, negotiation between staff and family much more explicit

staff able to be confrontational (where appropriate) with clients, talking about families in more realistic ways. (p. 42)

The managers also noted the beneficial effect on safe practice which had been achieved particularly in terms of working openly with families, record keeping and better report writing. One manager also thought a large number of staff felt 'safer' in their work.

Conclusions from evaluation of this project

Results obtained from evaluation of this project indicated that community nursing staff had been enabled and empowered in their child protection work by the presence of CPAs. The field staff felt they had been provided with advice and, importantly, support from their peers in a manner both appropriate and accessible, which had in turn greatly contributed to the development of their nursing practice in this area. A key feature within the above was the separation of supervision roles into the twin spheres of managerial and professional supervision. This in turn poses the larger question for debate of whether community nurse managers should continue to combine professional and managerial supervision in the future and, essentially, whether it is ever possible for them to do so.

One factor in addressing this question must surely be that of time — time to supervise staff in a *pro-active* not merely reactive manner. It is very easy for busy nurse managers with high workloads and multiple responsibilities and demands on their time to relegate supervision to a secondary and crisis-driven activity within their overall role. But can this then be described as supervision in any meaningful way? Or does it fulfil only the function of ensuring field staff work within the prescribed boundaries of agreed policies and procedures, rather than that other important and essential supervisory function of *actively* creating an environment in which staff are able to explore, analyze and develop their skills and practice with clients? The responsibilities of the professional supervisor are onerous, and as Hawkins and Shohat have said:

it is easy to use less structured types of supervision to avoid the rigours and concentrated focus of regular, formal individual sessions . . . It is easy to create a climate where supervision is only requested when you have a recognisable problem and at other times you have to be seen to 'soldier on'. (1989, p. 47)

Professional, pro-active supervision is certainly very costly in terms of time.

But surely field staff and their families have a right to, and deserve, such time, especially when one considers that time spent in this way can make the difference between *really* enabling change to take place within families and practitioners, and merely maintaining them just well enough to allow children to grow up without achieving their full potential and maybe even repeating the cycle of abuse?

A second factor within this debate must be that of the credibility of the supervisor in relation to staff she supervises. Can community nurse managers really claim to have up-to-date skills and expertise in clinical child protection work? Do they remember what it feels like to work in such a stressful situation, and do they have realistic expectations of their staff within this? An important point to bear in mind here is that for the member of staff who is perhaps experiencing difficulties in her work with an individual family, it may be tempting and relatively easy to disregard advice and support offered by a nurse manager in terms of 'she doesn't know what she's talking about' or 'she doesn't understand the context/situation/current practice issues'. The appointment of CPAs who also undertake clinical practice work automatically circumvents and negates such a response and also provides models of *actual* good practice which staff can then follow.

Thirdly, there is the question of how the supervision needs of nurse managers themselves are or can be met. Clearly, nurse managers who supervise community nurses in child protection work require both professional and managerial supervision.

Finally, and perhaps most fundamentally, there is also the factor concerning supervision as a means of monitoring individual staff performance, and supervision as a means of allowing staff to freely express their worries, anxieties and problems in relation to their current practice. These two elements of the supervision function can be contradictory in that staff will not necessarily want to reveal their innermost anxieties to their line manager who has a personnel function in respect of them. And yet they actually *need* to share and explore such concerns if they are to develop both personally and professionally. The professional supervisory role contains elements akin to that of both a confidante and a friend. On this it is useful to consider the widely held view that it is difficult for anyone to be 'good enough' parent without help and support. This provides a useful analogy for professional supervision in that the 'good enough' community nurse is enabled to survive negative or stressful experiences of child protection work through the strength of herself being held within, and by, the supervisory relationship.

The supervisor's role is not just to reassure the worker, but to allow the emotional disturbance to be felt within the safer setting of the supervisory relationship, where it can be survived, reflected upon and learnt from. Supervision thus provides a container that holds the helping relationship within the 'therapeutic triad'. (Hawkins and Shohat, 1989, p. 1)

Should the nurse manager take such issues on board, given that to do so may increase and/or emphasise a relationship of power between herself and her staff and, simultaneously, may also lead to a situation in which both managers and staff minimise the impact of any stress? I believe they should not and that it is beneficial to both nurse managers and community nursing staff to separate out the professional and managerial supervisory functions, since these contain elements of control and monitoring, and elements of facilitation and enablement, which, though both essential and important, can be experienced as a contradiction. Currently in the UK, supervision of nurses and health visitors in child protection work falls mainly within the parameters of managerial supervision. The debate over the differences between managerial and professional supervision for community nursing practice, and who can best meet those different needs, is long overdue.

The pilot child protection advisers project in Tower Hamlets Health Authority was evaluated as a resounding success by nurse managers, child protection advisers and community nurses. This scheme of organising child protection work and supervision therein has therefore continued to operate.

References

Department of Health and Social Security (1988) *Child Protection: Guidance for Senior Nurses, Health Visitors and Midwives.* London: HMSO.

Hawkins, P. and Shohat, R. (1989) *Supervision in the Helping Professions.* Milton Keynes: Open University Press.

Jones, D., Pickett, J., Oates, M. and Barbor, P. (1987) *Understanding Child Abuse.* 2nd edn. London: Macmillan.

London Borough of Greenwich and Greenwich Health Authority (1987) *Protection of Children in a Responsible Society.* London: London Borough of Greenwich.

North East Thames Regional Health Authority (1988) *Policy Statement on the Management of Child Abuse.* London: North East Thames Regional Health Authority.

Open University (1990) *Child Abuse and Neglect: An Introduction.* Milton Keynes: Open University Press.

Taket, A. et al. (1990) *Report on the Child Protection Advisers Project in Tower Hamlets.* London: Department of Geography, Queen Mary and Westfield College, University of London.

United Kingdom Central Council for Nurses, Midwives and Health Visitors (1989) *Code of Professional Conduct.* London: UKCC.

6 Communicating assertively to protect children in nursing practice

Peter Tattersall

A number of factors conspire to make communication in child protection difficult. Communication is affected by the power relations between the different professionals involved. There is also invariably an unequal relationship between the professionals and the parents and the children. Class, race, gender and professional and organisational structures all threaten open communication and clear thinking and as a result the safety and protection of children are jeopardised. Also important is how the individual feels about herself, how others perceive and respond to her, and what has been her past experience in communicating both in general and specifically over child protection matters.

If nurses and health visitors are to make high quality decisions about the wellbeing of children, they need to have all the relevant information available to them. For this reason it is vitally important that what the nurse thinks, believes and feels about a situation is communicated to appropriate others — workers, managers, parents and the children themselves — in an open, firm and respectful way: in other words, assertively.

The best interests of children demand that nurses and health visitors communicate their concerns to carers, to each other, and to other professionals, and that they assertively ask each other to express their concerns. Moreover, assertive communication not only makes for better practice, it also enhances the practitioner's confidence. Success will breed success.

This chapter considers what is meant by assertive communication, provides guidance on identifying past successes, and outlines strategies for building on them.

What assertive communication is — and what it is not

Any one situation will provoke a number of different responses, not all of which will be assertive. Consider the following statements:

- 'I am always right about these situations so I make sure I get decisions to go my way, even if it means stepping on a few toes in the process. I detest time-wasting discussions and I let people know it too.'
- 'I don't see any harm in not going into all the details, or embroidering some of them with a bit of emotion, it's the interests of the child I'm thinking about.'
- 'I say that I feel concerned but it doesn't seem to count for much so I don't like to push it, I'm not an expert after all.'
- 'I think about the causes of my concerns, then state them, as clearly and as fully as I can. I also encourage others to share their concerns so that we have the full picture.'

A range of child protection situations may provoke such responses, perhaps not least the case conference involving professionals from a number of disciplines. Which statement represents assertive thinking?

The first statement describes aggressive communication. This is the person who believes that a good decision is where everyone agrees with him and to achieve this he is prepared to bully, intimidate and talk down to others. The approach is 'open', but because it is disrespectful of other people's views it goes beyond firmness into aggression.

The second statement assumes that the way to get a good decision is to manipulate other people by withholding information or deliberately distorting it. This involves playing on other people's feelings to get them to agree. This person may be 'firm', but the lack of openness is certainly disrespectful of others.

The third statement represents a submissive communication. This person has allowed an earlier experience of not being listened to or understood to influence current communication. There is deference to the 'experts'. The individual does not expect to be listened to and the expectation is fulfilled because of it. This person may respect 'expert' opinions but she does not respect her own and this results in a lack of firmness.

The fourth statement *is* an assertive approach to communication. This person has prepared what she wants to say and has access to what she believes is the relevant information. She also sees her role as contributing to rather than necessarily 'winning' the argument and she is firm in ensuring her right to do so. The approach complies with the three criteria for assertive communication: it is open, firm and respectful.

Towards communicating assertively

In order to develop assertiveness skills it is valuable for you to identify past situations in which you expressed something you thought, believed or felt in an open, firm and respectful way. Consider the following questions:

- Who was the person or people you were communicating with?
- What was the situation?
- What did you want to say?
- How did you say it?
- How did they respond?
- How did you deal with their response?
- How did the conversation end?

From this, principles can be derived which could be applied to future situations. Consideration can also be given to successful practices which may be worth repeating. You could begin this process by completing the following sentences:

> *Principles*
> 'In future I will always . . .'
> 'In future I will never . . .'
>
> *Successful practices*
> 'I will repeat the following practice . . . when . . .'

It may also be valuable to start a log or diary of current situations, particularly if it is difficult to remember ones from the past. An *assertiveness communication diary* can facilitate continuous assessment and improvement of practice by enabling the logging of situations when they are fresh in the mind, including important details and subtleties which would otherwise be lost. In a busy day this may feel like a good but an impractical idea. In which case, make a brief and concise note either at the first opportunity — between visits or meetings — or at a particular time each day when you can have five minutes' thinking time.

In addition to the principles which are developed from your own practice, consider adding the following:

- Know your aims.
- Prepare for problems.
- Use personal authority.
- Work in partnership.
- Exercise your rights.
- Make plans to improve.

Your own principles will probably have much more meaning and value because you have 'lived' them. New principles should be added as they are discovered from new experiences.

What makes assertive communication a challenge?

Nurses, managers and employers make a number of assumptions about each other, and how they behave towards each other is a consequence of this. These assumptions have little to do with how individuals are seen as people but are more to do with how they are perceived as members of particular groups. Groups may be based on race, sex, class, physical ability, religion and lifestyle to name but a few. These assumptions can, when manifested in subtle or overt behaviours, undermine the individual's ability to be open, firm and respectful with others.

To communicate assertively, oppressive behaviour, practised both towards ourselves and by us, needs to be recognised and dealt with. This chapter can do little more than touch on a number of issues.

Racist assumptions affect how white people behave towards black people. Television and newspapers regularly portray black people as at best menial workers and at worst criminals. To take one of very many examples, the news media often report crimes which identify the race of the person only when they are black, even though this information is irrelevant to the criminal behaviour of the individual concerned. The effect, however, is to give a distorted picture which portrays black people as criminals. As a consequence many white people assume that most black people are in fact criminals and behave accordingly.

Sexist assumptions are endemic in society and also in the health service. Medicine is a predominantly male profession and nursing a female profession; doctors are paid substantially more than nurses and this is a reflection of the value placed by society on their role; the managers are overwhelmingly male and the managed female. The physical tasks of caring for patients are in the main carried out by women. In this way the sexism of wider society — inculcated from birth — is perpetuated through the institution of the health service. This is bound to affect how men and women relate to one another. It is easier to act according to the role prescribed by society than to challenge it.

Assumptions based on social class are widespread. Working-class people are often portrayed in a derogatory way — as stupid, inadequate, unsophisticated and sometimes as brutal. Conversely, owning and middle class people — their lifestyles, values and aspirations — are depicted in a very positive way. In the area of child protection, such views are apparent in the often expressed view — particularly propagated by the media — that child abuse is most widespread among the working class and that the middle classes and people who send their children away to boarding schools do not abuse and neglect their children. The reality, of course, is that child protection agencies, fuelled by such assumptions, look for child abuse on council estates where inadequate parenting is most visible. Because working class people as a whole are held in low esteem by society, this can and often does result in low personal esteem. This is reinforced through their experiences of people from other classes who act on society's assumptions, albeit unconsciously for the most part.

Equal opportunities legislation seeks to counter *assumptions based on physical ability*. People with disabilities are all too often accorded second class status and related to in terms of their disability rather than as people. The notion that 'deaf equals daft' is widespread. There is a fear of people who have a disability or a learning difficulty. One way of coping with the fear is to ignore it or minimise its importance. In child protection terms it is a major cause for concern that the signs and symptoms of children who have been abused are often ignored or attributed to their disability rather than to the trauma of the abuse which they have suffered.

Assumptions based on lifestyle will also affect professionals' behaviour. Lesbians and gay men are often assumed to be 'deviant' or 'immoral' because their lifestyle does not conform to the majority lifestyle of heterosexuals. The focus on homosexuals is often on the sexual act rather than on a loving relationship. This is in contrast to heterosexual couples, with whom the quality of their relationship and the type of people they are is the more usual interest. The pressure to conform is often violent, and makes it very difficult for lesbians and gay men to be open about who they really are.

In looking at these issues and linking them together it may be easy to draw the conclusion that it is the white, middle-class, able bodied, heterosexual men who are the 'bad people'. In fact the issue is less to do with bad and good people and more to do with oppressive and supportive behaviour. On a personal level, focusing on behaviour provides an opportunity to discourage the one and encourage the other by using assertive communication, and can help empower us to influence the people around us. This, however, has to be seen in the following contexts.

Professional status

Two challenges for nurses and health visitors posed at the professional level are to do with status: the status of other professionals and the status of the information they provide.

Because doctors and some other professionals around the case conference table are sometimes perceived to have more professional status than nurses and health visitors, this can make it more difficult for the latter to be heard. 'High status' professionals are likely to be given even higher status if they also happen to be men. In reality, health visitors and nurses have many advantages over their colleagues, deriving from their work and the relationship and rapport which they are able to establish with families.

Medical information is accorded higher status than other types of information — in part because it is perceived as more 'scientific' and is also harder to question without expert knowledge. Conversely, information which is based on intuitive feelings, resulting from observations and reactions to the relationship between the child and the parent or carer is much more easily questioned, even if it is thought valuable in the first place.

However, it is not ethical or desirable to medically examine every child who has contact with the health service for abuse. Nor is it the case any longer that medical opinions based on physical examination are beyond dispute, as the Cleveland Inquiry has shown. When this is coupled with the fact that the initial concerns often rely on 'social' rather than medical information, it becomes all the more unacceptable that social information is given a lower status.

High-quality child protection decisions thus rely on all the people involved assertively stating their concerns and actively and assertively requesting this of each other.

The challenge of child protection

A constant challenge in child protection is denial and over-reaction. There is a tendency for professionals to deny that there is any real problem, when sometimes there really is. Some of the feelings which lead professionals to look for reassurance that everything is all right are: a fear that the relationship with the child's carer will be damaged if questions are asked; anxiety about taking on yet another case when resources are already stretched; and an unwillingness to believe that a carer has deliberately caused significant harm to a child. All of this can subconsciously result in a reduction of appropriate concern and an acceptance of the carer's denials. The professional will find it much more emotionally comfortable to be reassured by a justification of excuse, than to confront the possibility that the child is indeed at risk.

When and if concerns do then bubble up to the surface it can often produce the opposite effect — over-reaction. This can send professionals into a frenzied panic, in which thinking becomes muddled and reactive, and more extreme measures and actions are taken than are necessary. The professional's behaviour is then not appropriate to the time and stage of the identification of the abuse. It is a swing from the passive behaviour of denial to the aggressive behaviour of over-reaction, driven by fear and anger.

Using assertive communication in child protection

The following child protection cameos describe how Barbara, a health visitor, deals with three situations. Because she finds them particularly difficult, she is unable to be as assertive as she might be and is therefore unhappy with the way things turn out. In reading the cases, imagine what Barbara could have done differently and what you would have done if you were the health visitor.

Cameo: The Social Services referral

Barbara has been working with a young mother and her baby. The mother has been in long-term residential care and is now living in a home which helps young people leave care and live independently. One afternoon, the mother's partner arrives at the home drunk and is rude and aggressive towards the mother and the staff. The home telephones the mother's social worker, Phillip, to tell them of their concerns.

Barbara receives a phone call from Phillip, who asks her to visit the partner and assess the risk to the baby from this person. Barbara explains that this is not her role as a health visitor, says she feels it is inappropriate for her to visit and politely says no.

Later that day, Barbara receives a call from her manager, a senior nurse, who says that the Social Services Department does not have the resources to visit the partner and that Barbara will have to make the visit. She adds that she is very worried about the safety of this baby and cannot stop thinking about what might happen if the partner arrives in a drunken state again. Barbara reluctantly agrees.

From then on she constantly finds herself being asked to do things which are not really part of her job.

Comment It would seem that, for some reason Barbara's manager was unable to be assertive with Phillip. Had she been assertive, she would have repeated Barbara's position to Phillip, resulting in him taking responsibility for his area of work. As a consequence of not doing so, she was left having to persuade Barbara to make the visit to the partner. She achieved this partly by inappropriately using her authority as a manager, but more effectively by manipulating Barbara's feelings — the underlying message is 'I won't be able to stop worrying unless you do this for me.' It is a very powerful message which prevented Barbara making an assertive statement like 'I understand how worried you are about the baby. However, it is not my job to visit. If Phillip has a resource problem, he should take it to his manager for a decision, not to you. I would like to help but it really is quite inappropriate for me to do so.'

Cameo: the home visit

Barbara visits a mother and her toddler at home one day to discover that the child appears to be in some pain. The mother, when asked about this, says he fell against the radiator and burnt his neck.

Barbara asks the mother to show her the burns and does not think that these are the type that a hot radiator would make. She is pretty sure that the burns were caused by something else. However, because Barbara is developing a good relationship with this mother who has always been a bit touchy and uncomfortable with her in the past, she is worried about exploring it any further in case the mother rejects her. She would then feel she had failed in this piece of work and would not have the opportunity to help the mother take better care of the baby.

Although she is extremely concerned about the burns she decides to accept the explanation and see if she can give her a bit more time and support in the future.

Comment Barbara is allowing her fears of upsetting the parent and the possibility of losing her relationship with her to dictate her behaviour. In fact the converse may be true. It may well be that if she does not confront her, the mother may lose respect for Barbara because she knows she can say anything and be believed. Barbara has to see the relationship with the mother as a partnership which exists for the best interests of the child. That means asking awkward, difficult and uncomfortable questions about the child's welfare when something appears to be wrong.

To do this assertively, Barbara needs to ask straightforwardly for more information to help her understand how the child received the burns. 'Did you see it happen? Which radiator did he fall against? How did he come to fall over? How long do you think his neck was against the radiator? How hot was the radiator? Was he wearing anything around his neck at the time?'

This assertive questioning will either support the mother's account of, if not, provide the basis for the next assertive communication — 'I really can't understand how he got these burns from the radiator in the way that you describe. I am very concerned that he may have been burned in some other way. Is there anything else you would like to tell me?'

This may prompt the mother to disclose the real cause of the burns. If she insists on the original explanation, Barbara would need to say in a non-judgemental way that she suspects the burn is a non-accidental injury. She will then need to outline her professional responsibility to follow up her concerns and what this will mean in practical terms.

Cameo: the case conference

Barbara is at a case conference which is discussing a baby who has been burned by a cigarette. Round the table are: the mother and her new partner, a psychologist, a doctor, a teacher, a senior social worker who is chairing the conference, and the baby's social worker. The only other professional in the room that Barbara knows is Helen, the social worker. Unfortunately, she is in complete disagreement with Helen's assessment of the situation. She also dislikes the way that Helen is always rushing around in a panic, unable to focus on any one thing for very long.

Helen, when asked by the chair to give her assessment, refers to her file and says that in her opinion the mother has previously been unstable but is now stabilising due to the influence of her new partner. Helen smiles at the family and they smile back. She explains that the cigarette burn was a regrettable accident but that does not cause her any concern for the future.

Barbara, who is sitting back from the table with her arms crossed and looking at the edge of the table, is invited to comment. She says that she is worried about the cigarette burn and thinks that there is reason to be concerned. She would like to say why but suddenly feels it would be uncomfortable to do so in front of the family, and she finds herself unable to say anything or indeed look up from the table.

The chair asks Barbara what she proposes should be done about her concerns. Taken by surprise at this, she looks up at the ceiling for a moment to think, and then, addressing an empty space a foot to the right of the chair's shoulder, says she thinks she needs some

support. Helen guffaws and says: 'That's typical of a health visitor.'
Barbara shrinks even further back into her chair and studies the floor
intensely.

Consequently, the conference accepts the social worker's assessment and the child is considered not to be at risk. Eight months later
the baby is admitted to hospital with some serious non accidental
injuries. Helen has been on long term sick leave for the past five
months.

Comment Barbara was unprepared for the conference and was
consequently unable to assertively present her case. She did not have
her file with her and so could not use her notes to help her put her case
across. She also had not anticipated how it would feel to criticise the
parents to the conference in their presence, and so think about how
she might voice her concerns.

She had not thought in detail about what she would propose if she
had persuaded the conference to share her concerns. Support from
who, to do what, for how long, with what result? This led to the 'put
down' by Helen from which Barbara shrank instead of confronting it.

The messages she communicated with her body were also
unassertive. Sitting back from the table suggests to other people she
does not really want to be at the conference and would prefer to
remain passive. Her folded arms suggest that she is not 'open' to
anything anyone has to say because she has already made up her mind.
She avoided eye contact with anyone, preferring to look down, up or
to the side of the people to whom she was talking. This suggested she
was unconfident about her concerns and conclusions.

Techniques for communicating assertively

In child protection work there are a number of important circumstances in which nurses and health visitors need to act and communicate assertively. A number of techniques may be used and developed
in order to facilitate assertive communication and some of these are
described below.

Know your aims

The ability to communicate assertively increases proportionately with
how well the individual defines her aims. It is useful to give some
thought to the following three levels of questions in advance of a
meeting, visit, discussion or conference:

1   Why am I concerned about this child?
    What benefit can I be to this child in my professional role?

What do I need to say and do about my concerns and to whom?
2   What position do I want to be in by the end of this conversation?
    What do I need to have by the end of this discussion?
3   How will I know if I am successful in protecting this child?
    What must people have said, done or agreed to, for me to feel the discussion has been successful?

In other words, identify aims and plan accordingly. In the last cameo situation of the case conference, Barbara had not thought through her aims.

Prepare for problems

Barbara had not thought about how difficult it would be to criticise the parents in their presence. The individual nurse may have quite a good idea of people with whom she finds it difficult to be assertive. It is helpful to consciously think about who in particular these are. They could be:

- the child's siblings/parents/carers/relatives, and the child
- other nurses
- professional colleagues — doctors, social workers, psychologists, police
- the individual line manager
- other managers
- others.

Having identified the individuals with whom communication is difficult, it is then helpful to establish what *sorts of communication* are difficult with that person or people. These include:

- giving praise
- receiving praise
- stating an unpopular opinion
- raising difficulties
- responding to criticisms
- making requests
- saying 'no'.

Each of these is discussed in turn.
Giving praise   If you genuinely appreciate or agree with what someone is doing or saying, then praising her lets her know how you feel. This can be a powerful motivator and the person is much more likely to act in the same way again. It may also increase the person's willingness to co-operate with you in the future.
However, praising is not a common practice in white British

culture and it can feel awkward giving praise, even if you are used to it in another culture. The type of praise given is important but distinctions should be made. For example, it can be quite risky to give unspecific praise, like saying to a parent 'You're a good mother'. This can arouse suspicion because people often experience unspecific praise as a preface to being asked for something. In other words, the praise is being used in a manipulative way. If the person is able to accept praise they will feel good for a while and then forget about it. And the more times you say it, the less effect it will have.

Much safer and more effective praise is that which is specific to what you appreciate or approve of about the person. For example, 'You're very good at comforting your baby when he is upset — you pick him up straightaway.' This praises the mother in a way which tells her exactly what you think she is doing which is effective.

Although specific praise is more difficult because it requires you to use skills in observing effective practices, it is far more useful. It enables you to reinforce behaviours you want others to repeat. Because people on the whole enjoy being valued in this way they may be more willing to co-operate with you in the future. It can also improve their motivation because they will know that you are likely to notice if they are doing something useful or particularly well.

Moreover, when it becomes necessary to raise some difficulties with someone, she is much more likely to be able to respond assertively if she has been valued. Giving praise on a regular basis goes a long way to building a strong relationship.

Receiving praise can feel embarrassing and uncomfortable if you are unused to it. You may try to discount praise or diminish it in some way. Praise may come from colleagues, managers and indeed from families with whom the nurse is working. It may be particularly difficult accepting praise from families, because the praise may be construed as the mother crossing a professional barrier and the nurse may feel that such comments are either unwarranted or that they are so rare that they come as a complete surprise.

It is helpful to practise accepting praise when it is given and even agreeing with it. The other person should be thanked for the praise as it will encourage her to act in such a way again.

Stating an unpopular opinion can be extremely difficult, for example, as at a case conference. This is because it can get tangled up in wanting to feel approved of and popular as a nurse or health visitor. Before you voice your opinion you may feel increasingly tense and anxious, question your own ability, and feel critical towards other people. This is a natural and common reaction.

These feelings become more of a problem if they become bottled up to the extent that you feel ready to explode. If left to the actual situation you will probably have one of two reactions: either repressing your feelings and behaving passively for fear of stating your opinion too strongly, or being unable to contain your feelings and expressing yourself in short, aggressive bursts. Either way, you will not be communicating your opinion assertively.

If you can, find some time to express these feelings before the event. You could ask a friend or colleague to represent the other people while you just 'let off steam' and they listen. What you should say is the 'feelings' version which may well be rude or impolite, not what you actually intend to say. Your friend's role is to smile and invite you to be even ruder, angrier, or whatever else it is you are feeling. Then, in the real situation, there is a better chance that your feelings will be in proportion to the situation and you can express them more appropriately.

In addition, preparing what you are going to say and how you will say it, will greatly assist you in assertively stating your opinion. One approach is to write this down and rehearse it with a colleague or friend so that when the time comes to state it, your message is clear, brief, to the point, and purposeful. Follow this by making some plans to assertively respond to objections. Use your fantasies of what people might say to identify likely objections and plan your answers to them.

However, beware of procrastination. Nurses and health visitors face heavy workloads and this, coupled with these difficult feelings can lead to putting off preparation. You can find yourself doing all those little jobs you suddenly discover have to be done just right now and so you run out of time. Do not allow your fears to undermine your effectiveness — put aside time in your diary to prepare and guard it preciously.

There are a number of techniques which will help you communicate assertively in any situation, not least when you wish to state an unpopular opinion:

- Keep eye contact with the people and break it every four or five seconds to avoid staring.
- Sit or stand upright so that you are not leaning inwards in an aggressive stance or backwards in a retreating, passive stance.
- Keep your arms to the side of your body in an open, welcoming gesture, with your fingers loosely curled, not in fists.
- Say 'I believe' or 'I think' rather than 'It is believed' or other statements which disown the opinion.
- Say what you have to say as clearly, concisely and briefly as possible.
- Invite and welcome questions.

By following these suggestions there is a better chance that your opinion will be taken seriously, leading to proper discussion and

consideration. If this then influences the outcome in a way that you
approve of, so much the better. If not, then the important thing is that
you are satisfied that your opinion has been aired.

Listening to and exploring an unpopular opinion is an important
part of assertive communication. A natural reaction to an opinion with
which you strongly disagree is either to ignore it, which is a passive
response, or to attack it, an aggressive response. In so doing the
opportunity to reaffirm your opinion or to change your mind in the
light of new information may be missed. In these sorts of situation it
may be helpful to:

- hear what the person has to say. That means no interrupting
  them, and making a careful mental or written note of what
  exactly they are saying. Strong feelings impair the ability to
  listen accurately.
- ask questions to clarify exactly what is being said and what is
  not.
- ask why the person thinks the way they do.
- apply their thinking to other situations and see if the logic
  holds true.
- decide whether they have a point and accept it if they do.
- if you disagree, say so, firmly and with reasons.

Nursing practice will provide many opportunities in which nurses and
health visitors have to listen to opinions with which they disagree.
These will include encounters with both parents and carers and also
professionals from other disciplines.

Strategies need to be developed for *raising difficulties*. It is always
worth thinking twice if you are tempted to blame, attack or criticise
another person. if you do not like what another person is doing, then
it is probably more effective to think about how you might help them
to do it differently rather than 'have a go at them'. This is not easy
because, the more you dislike what they are doing the more hostile
you will feel and the less likely you will be able to raise the difficulty in
a supportive way. The following suggestions may be helpful:

- Consider whether it really matters if you dislike what the
  person is doing, for example, not putting baby to bed at the
  same time every night if baby is actually getting enough sleep.
- If it matters very much and you have strong feelings, either tell
  someone else how you feel first, to get it off your chest, or write
  down your feelings. Then you can think more clearly about
  how you can tell the person assertively.
- Speak to the person in private so that they do not feel they are
  losing face in front of others. With an audience, they will
  attack you to avoid losing face, rather than consider what you
  are saying.

- Be open about your feelings without blaming the other person for them — for example, understand the difference between saying 'When you do that, I feel anxious, concerned and angry . . .' rather than 'You make me feel anxious . . .'
- Be specific about any concerns you have without judging the person. Rather than say 'Don't leave the fire unguarded, you're being really irresponsible', say 'If you leave the fire unguarded then Yvonne will probably burn herself, she's too young to know how dangerous it is.'

Given that blame, attack and criticism are not assertive behaviours and are unlikely to help a situation, there is a choice about your *response to criticisms* of you.

If the criticism is very strong you would be within your rights to just simply and firmly interrupt with a statement such as 'You are talking to me in an unacceptable/sexist/racist way and I refuse to listen to it.'

If the criticism is milder, you chould choose to change the tone of it by:

- asking the person to say more about what they do not like
- requesting them to leave out any personal comments and instead focus on your behaviour — what you have done and said
- inviting them to say how they think you should do things differently in future
- if you disagree saying either 'I understand how you feel but I'm afraid I'm not prepared to change what I do' or say 'I'll think about it and come back and let you know what I have decided to do.'
- if you agree, accepting their point politely and reaching an agreement about how you will do things differently in future.

By changing the tone in this way you are inviting them to help you look at the situation and to think about it.

Working in partnership with parents and professionals will mean *making requests* of each other in order to protect children. As in any relationship where there is a mutual dependence to achieve common goals, working together requires people to contribute their ideas, skills, information and expertise.

Sometimes making a request can be difficult. You may feel guilty about asking a busy person to do yet something else. You may feel another person may not do the job properly and you would be better off doing it yourself. If you act on these feelings, they will undermine your ability to work as an equal partner with others. Partnerships are built on people doing things for each other for mutual benefit.

If you feel awkward about making a request, take a moment to consider why and see if you recognise any of these feelings. If you have childhood experiences which deter you, recognise them for what they are and that you needed to act in this way to get by as a child. As an adult you can choose to do things differently despite feeling awkward.

Busy people are often used to handling a heavy workload. If you feel guilty about asking them remember that they can always say 'no'. If they really cannot handle it, they do have a choice.

The fear that if you ask somebody for something they will not do it properly is common and understandable. Use this feeling to help you work out what exactly you would need if it were done to your standards. When you then make your request you can be very specific about what you want. If you make a very 'open' request, you will get an 'open' response, i.e. not necessarily the result you had in mind. Be as clear and specific as possible.

Saying 'yes' to someone is far easier than *saying 'no'* because that is what they want you to say. However, the warm feelings that come from their gratitude can quickly be replaced with feelings of panic, resentment or regret: 'How on earth am I going to find the time?', 'Why should I do it?' or 'Actually, I don't agree.'

You might also feel obliged to agree if the person is your manager, has some authority within their profession, or is someone to whom you give a lot of authority. However, you are by no means obliged to do everything anyone tells you just because they have some authority. Your agreement should be dependent on whether their request is reasonable and appropriate, and on what are the risks and gains of agreeing or disagreeing.

In one of the cameo illustrations, the health visitor reluctantly agreed to her manager's request to visit a family and undertake a risk assessment despite feeling it was not her role to do so.

The important thing is to listen to your feelings when you first receive the request, not afterwards when you have committed yourself. Listen to your feelings, think it over for a few seconds and then reply. If you need more time to consider you can always say 'I'll come back to you on that', as long as you say when you will let them know and make sure that you do it.

If you do decide to say 'no', give your reasons. If the person persists in asking, then you may have to just keep repeating your explanation. Avoid adding or inventing new reasons — they will not be as strong as your original statement and you may find yourself giving in. Some people need to hear the same thing several times before they accept it.

In saying 'no', it can sometimes help to empathise by saying something like 'I do understand that you've got a problem here, and I hope you can get someone to help you out.' This will let the person know that, although you are not giving them what they want, it is not because you do not care or are unsympathetic. This is far more effective than being over-apologetic and saying 'sorry' repeatedly. Saying 'sorry' may make you feel as if you have done something wrong or made a mistake. You have not, you are only saying 'no'.

If you really feel you cannot say 'no' without worse consequences than saying 'yes', then you can always set some limits — 'OK, but I can only do it for half an hour', for example. In this way, you are not saying 'no', but you are making it more manageable for yourself.

Use of personal authority

Authority is the ability to influence the outcome of events. People obtain authority in a number of ways: by rising up the hierarchy, by having expert knowledge, or by using personal authority in working with others. By learning to communicate more assertively, you are developing and increasing your personal authority. You are investing in yourself for life, not just in your current job, and will find that by being successful you will want to continue to be even more successful. Through experience will come the confidence to use this authority.

Taking personal authority means going beyond your own aims and personal perspectives and developing the ability to see the whole situation. Standing back and looking at the whole picture gives you a lot of valuable information about what should happen to improve things. To get the whole picture you need everyone's thoughts, feelings, knowledge and concerns. The best way to do that is to work in partnership with them. That is the basis of the case conference and, as was illustrated in one of the cameos, teamwork is not always easy, and it will almost certainly benefit from the team acting assertively.

Working in partnership

An effective outcome for a child is jeopardised if professionals act as individuals whose individual and professional pride is at stake. The danger in the individualist approach is that a key concern or piece of information that is held by someone is never heard. The one concern that would lead to a rational outcome is lost in a battle of individuals each seeking to get their own way or minimise loss of face.

If you see the parents and professionals with whom you are working as problem solving partners, rather than as opponents who have to be defeated, you can begin to work as a team in partnership. Working in partnership means being open to everyone's views and concerns in the early stages and being confident enough to rigorously assess all this information in order to arrive at a quality decision. It requires you to notice when people are not contributing and encourage them to do so, even if you do not always agree with the views that are being put forward or particularly like the people expressing them as people. It means being prepared to change your mind if new information comes to light which changes things. It also means believing that you are an effective professional whether or not others accept what you say about a particular child.

Partnership is the process of pooling resources and energy for the benefit of all the people in the partnership in order to make the most effective decision. Your contribution is essential to the process and you have every right to contribute as an equal and respected partner.

Exercise your rights

If you are prepared to work in partnership with others, then it is only reasonable to expect others to enter into the same spirit of co-operation. The following set of rights may help you recognise when a partnership is becoming one sided:

- You have the right to respect from others.
- You have the right to contribute from your special professional position as a nurse or health visitor.
- You have the right to your feelings, both negative and positive, and to express them openly.
- You have the right to express your concerns, opinions, beliefs and values.
- You have a right to change your mind.
- You have the right to say 'no'.
- You have a right to make requests of others.
- You have the right to object to and interrupt criticisms and personal abuse.
- You have the right to use your personal authority regardless of whether you are the designated 'leader' or not.
- You have the right to be successful, to make mistakes, and to learn from both.

Making plans to improve child protection practice

Assertive communication will enhance the practitioner's ability to protect children. This chapter has outlined a number of strategies which will help the nurse or health visitor communicate in the highly charged area of child protection work. It will be beneficial to identify the people and situations with whom and in which you find it difficult to be assertive and then apply some of the techniques which have been described in this chapter. There may be a number of such people or situations. These should then be ranked and you should seek to tackle the least difficult first since your chances of success will be greatest and your increased confidence will help you deal with the more difficult situations. Having identified the person or situation you wish to tackle, write down the following details:

- the name of the person and their relationship with you
- the situation which is particularly difficult
- the feelings you have identified in these situations
- ideas to make strong feelings manageable in advance of the situation
- what you would like to change about the way in which you communicate with this person and why
- what you are going to try out to see if it makes a difference
- the date, time and place the plan will be put into action (transfer into your diary).

As soon after the event as possible you will need to review how the plan went, noting which things went successfully and what did not seem to work so well. On the basis of that exercise, identify one or two things which you will repeat or do differently next time. You can then begin to plan for that next encounter.

Effective personal, professional and group planning is critical to effective child protection. Situations involving child abuse, almost by definition, generate a complex set of relationships and the individual nurse or health visitor — as with professionals from other disciplines — will find responding both challenging and emotionally demanding. Assertiveness skills and training will help equip the nurse for dealing with these difficult situations. However, it should not be forgotten that no matter how assertive an individual is, in child protection there may still be powerful forces beyond the control of any one person. The most assertive of people may be defeated by these forces, which may derive from social structures, wider ideologies, and systems of power. These wider forces have a profound impact on practice, and while assertiveness skills will not necessarily eliminate their impact, they will help the individual practise more effectively.

Further reading and resources

Brennan, Rosemary and Simmons, Michael, *United We Stand Divided We Fall: the Different Kinds of Oppression*. Institute for a New Leadership Initiative. Article.

Dickson, Anne, *A Woman in Your Own Right*, London: Quartet Books.

Fritchie, Rennie, *Working with Assertiveness*, BBC Training Video.

Janner, Carl and Thatcher, Basil, *The Motley Crew*. Video Arts. Video (with booklet).

Johnson, Clifford, *Assertiveness*. Sterling Professional Video (with booklet).

Acknowledgement

The author wishes to express his great appreciation to Isobel Bremmer, social worker and partner, for her excellent ideas and suggestions.

7 The construction of child abuse in the accident and emergency department

Jane Wynne

Nursing and other staff working in accident and emergency departments have a key role to play in identifying children who may have been abused and in initiating protective action. Recognition of child abuse is not always straightforward, and in the busy and pressurised world of the accident and emergency department cases may be missed. Accident and emergency nurses need to understand and be able to recognise indicators of child abuse, know what procedures to follow, and feel part of a wider team of professionals involved in child protection.

This chapter describes the broad context in which different types of child abuse occur and traces the history of the recognition of child abuse in hospital settings. Signs and symptoms of child abuse and neglect are outlined and the role of nursing staff, in response, is discussed, including action taken in supporting the children and their families.

Clinical practice in the recognition and management of child abuse has changed over the last thirty years. In the 1960s professionals in the accident and emergency department were at the forefront in the diagnosis of the 'battered baby syndrome' (Kempe et al., 1962). Grievously injured or dead babies were brought to the hospital. The infant had been shaken, swung by the legs against the wall, and there were injuries to match. Extensive bruising, multiple fracturing of skull, long bones, ribs, retinal haemorrhages and subdural haematoma were found on examination clinically, radiologically and at autopsy.

Seriously injured babies are still seen today, but, with the recognition of the significance of more minor injuries, the numbers of severely injured babies declined over the next twenty years. This trend may now be altering once again.

Physical abuse may begin as physical punishment (however inappropriate) and escalates, as it proves ineffective, to beating. A better understanding of the relationship between physical punishment and child abuse is only recent (Newell, 1989). The Newsons (1965) showed that the British are a nation of hitters and smackers. Ninety-seven per cent of four-year-old children are hit, the majority between one and six times each week. Prevention of child abuse is a complex issue, but the work of EPOCH demonstrating alternative ways of child-rearing without resorting to physical violence is an important step forward.

Current statistics on child abuse do not give any grounds for complacency. The numbers and percentages of children registered with fatal and serious injury increased between 1983 and 1987, the last year for which NSPCC figures are available at the time of writing, from 0.06 per thousand children in 1983 to 0.13 in 1987 (Creighton and Noyes, 1989). The NSPCC estimates that 150–200 children die in England and Wales each year from the effects or consequences of child abuse and neglect. Many of these deaths go unrecognised as due to child maltreatment. The recent Department of Health figures (1991a) showed a 6 per cent increase in the number of children on child protection registers from 1989 to 1990, or 4 per 1000 children of the population under the age of eighteen years on register in England. This is a total of approximately 43,600 children. The breakdown of registrations concerning abused children in the Department of Health statistics are: 27 per cent non-accidental injury, 15 per cent sexual abuse and 41 per cent grave concern.

Whether the increased numbers of parents attending child protection conferences will affect the rate of registration of children will be an important trend to observe. Likewise, the category 'grave concern' is no longer available to conferences and this may affect registration rates too.

The Children Act will directly influence the management of child abuse. The current guidance for inter-agency working, *Working Together*, is subtitled *under the Children Act 1989*. These guidelines 'should be complied with unless local circumstances indicate exceptional reasons which justify variation' (Department of Health, 1991b). Clearly, the status of *Working Together* should be noted.

Three important themes of management are:

1   There should be a partnership with families throughout child protection procedures.
2   Child protection procedures apply universally and thus include foster homes, children's homes and boarding schools.
3   Action taken should be decisive, rather than precipitative, to protect children from child abuse or neglect. The potential for damage to the long-term future of the child by precipitative action must be considered.

While it is essential to stop and think, and to discuss with colleagues any difficult points in management, it is also necessary to protect children. Families are not always reasonable, do not take responsibility and may be very difficult 'partners'. In the midst of our endeavours to engage families in positive work, the focus must remain on the child and his or her needs.

Poverty is a major stress in families. 'Good enough' parenting becomes more and more problematic in financially impoverished highly stressed families. There is a clear correlation between stress (marital, housing problems, low income) and physical abuse and neglect. It is much more difficult to rear children without the advantages of a good income and education. Large families and lone-parent families are the two groups who are the poorest in the UK, and many children are brought up on the boundaries of, or in, poverty. The origins of childhood poverty require urgent governmental attention.

Emotional abuse and child sexual abuse differ from physical abuse in that they are more evenly spread through the social strata and less related to social disadvantage.

Child sexual abuse has become a major social concern in the UK since the mid-1980s. The first and most widely reported inquiry into sexual abuse in the UK began its final conclusion:

> We have learned during the Inquiry that sexual abuse occurs in children of all ages, including the very young, to boys as well as girls in all classes of society and frequently within the privacy of the family. The sexual abuse can be very serious and on occasion include vaginal, anal and oral intercourse . . . (Butler-Sloss, 1988)

The NSPCC figures show that in 1983 60 per cent of registrations were because of physical abuse and 5 per cent because of sexual abuse, but by 1987 the respective figures were 35 per cent and 28 per cent (Creighton and Noyes, 1989).

In Leeds over half the referrals to paediatricians because of possible abuse are because of possible child sexual abuse (CSA). This involves 500–600 children each year out of a total number of around

1000 children referred. During the early 1980s in Leeds a diagnosis of probable child sexual abuse was made in ten or so children. The current rate of diagnosis of probable CSA is 250–300 children a year.

Emotional abuse is common; in all cases of child maltreatment there is an element of emotional abuse. In the absence of other abuses, emotional abuse is rarely diagnosed, yet it is probably the most common form of child maltreatment. In 1987 only 1 per cent of the total children registered were in the category of emotional abuse (Creighton and Noyes, 1989).

Where are abused children seen?

Another change which is relevant to the accident and emergency (A&E) department is where the abused children are seen. Historically, many physically abused children have been seen in accident and emergency departments and sexually abused children in police stations. This latter practice in particular has been deplored. The Cleveland Report commented: 'the child should be medically examined in a suitable and sensitive environment, where there are suitably trained staff available' (Butler-Sloss, 1988). Police stations are not suitable, and neither is the A&E department, which is often noisy, bustling and lacking in privacy, unless there is a separate children's A&E. Even then, there needs to be an area where children may play, parents have space and there are one or two interview rooms available with appropriately trained staff to care for the child and family. These conditions are not available in many A&E departments, and increasingly children are seen by arrangement by community paediatricians in the paediatric out-patient clinic or its equivalent.

Children and families will usually receive a better service if the appointment is planned and the child does not have to compete with ill patients, accident victims and so on. This is possible in the majority of cases, although physically abused and some sexually abused children require a same-day appointment. Hence the average A&E department should now receive fewer children who may have been abused, but the cases they do see will be 'difficult' ones who present indirectly. It is here that experience is invaluable, and the permanent nursing staff in A&E departments will often be the first to recognise abuse for what it is.

The experienced ambulance man may also realise that 'something is wrong' and pass on to the nursing staff his anxiety.

Clinical situations which should raise the question of abuse

The majority of parents attending the A&E department with their child are straightforward and open: the child has an injury or is ill. When should the receiving nurse be concerned?

The *presentation of the history* may give clues:

- Does the history make sense?
- What does the child say?
- Has there been a delay in seeking help?
- Have there been previous attendances at A&E?
- Is the history compatible with the child's development level?
- Have there been other health problems, scalds, failure to thrive?

The following case history is an illustration:

A baby of five months was found by his granny not to be moving his left leg. The leg looked swollen, movement was painful and x-ray showed a recent spiral fracture of the femur and two healing fractured ribs.

Commentary In the absence of bony disease (very rare) long bones do not fracture spontaneously. There must therefore be a history, in this case denied, help was not sought by the parents, and skeletal survey revealed bony injuries. A skeletal survey was essential and showed the severity of the abuse, what was a recent and what an old injury.

The *physical examination* must be detailed and include:

- a description of the presenting injury
- other injuries (e,g, torn frenulum, bruised ear)
- signs of neglect
- signs of growth delay, taking account of height, weight, head circumference and mid-upper circumference (measurements should be related to percentile charts)
- signs of sexual assault (see below).

Further medical investigations are needed in some instances:

- if the child is badly bruised, he should be examined for a bleeding or clotting disorder
- a bruised infant or toddler should usually have a skeletal survey (the young child cannot give a history of pain, limitation of use of limb etc.)
- if a child has one fracture, possibly due to abuse, the need for a skeletal survey should always be considered, even in an older child.

Injuries of certain types should always alert staff to the possibility of abuse:

- fracture under the age of two years, and certainly under one year (Worlock et al., 1986)
- multiple fracture (metaphyseal, long bones, ribs)
- rib fractures (rare except in road traffic accidents)
- skull fracture — multiple, depressed, wide, long, growing (Hobbs, 1984)
- any bruising in infancy
- bruises to ears, cheek, lower jaw, neck, chest, back (Robertson et al., 1982).

Scalds and burns may also be the result of inflicted injury or lapses in protection of the child from danger. This form of abuse is under-recognised but there are indications:

- Is the scald recent, or has there been delay in seeking help?
- Is the scale on the shoulder and upper chest usual when a child pulls a cup of hot tea over himself?
- If the scalds are on his *buttocks, back* of the hands, *soles* of the feet, how did these occur? (Hobbs, 1986)
- Are the scalds in glove or stocking distribution, i.e. is this a forced immersion?

A *differential diagnosis* should be considered for bruising, fractures or skin lesions but, given a careful history and appropriate investigation, disease may usually be differentiated from congenital abnormality or trauma (Wheeler & Hobbs, 1988). Table 7.1 gives examples:

Table 7.1

Disorder	Investigation
Multiple bruises? idiopathic thrombocytopenia purpura (ITP)	Blood count — low platelet count — ITP
Multiple bruises? Clotting disorder, e.g. haemophilia	Prolonged partial thromboplastin time, Factor VIII level low — haemophilia
Multiple purple marks, back, buttocks, lower limb? Mongolian blue spot	Marks all same colour, do not change with time (thus not bruises) = Mongolian blue spot
Multiple fractures in infancy (Taitz, 1988) a) ? Osteogenesis imperfecta b) ? Copper deficiency in ex-premature baby — rare unless IV or other unusual feeding	a) Family history, blue sclerae. X-ray abnormality b) Low copper level, low [Caeruloplasmin] Hypochromic, microcytic anaemia

Munchausen Syndrome by proxy is a disorder of particular importance in A&E departments. Most departments know their 'adult regulars' who present with fictitious illness. It is more difficult to recognise the very concerned mother who repeatedly returns with the infant, complaining the child suffers from apnoea attacks or unexplained episodes of drowsiness. As all attendances of children aged up to sixteen years at A&E departments should now be passed on to the child's health visitor and general practitioner (DoH, 1991b), repeated attendance should be recognised. Clinically, once the possibility of fictitious illness has been raised, admission to a paediatric unit is needed. This is the only way the complex and serious cases may be unravelled, although there are no doubt many, many more minor cases currently of children attending GPs surgeries or paediatric out-patient clinics with fictitious fevers, fits or skin disorders. The most dangerous clinical situations are in the younger children and especially babies with breathing problems.

Deliberate poisoning or *suffocations* differ in some respects from Munchausen-by-proxy in that this may be a single act of violence towards the child rather than a prolonged 'illness' inflicted upon him.

In all unconscious children, fitting children or apnoeic children the possibility of poisoning and suffocation should be considered. This includes Sudden Infant Death Syndrome which clearly calls for a very high level of sensitivity and clinical skill in order not to add to the distress of anguished parents (Newlands and Emery, 1991).

Neglect is evident in the general physical state of the child. When the child is undressed and weighed note should be taken of

- his clothing — appropriate, thin, dirty?
- his body — dirty, scratched, bruised? Is there nappy rash?
- his hair — matted, thin? Is there cradle-cap?
- his nails — thickened, yellow?
- his teeth — not cleaned? Are there caries?
- his height and weight (refer to percentile chart)
- his behaviour — apathetic, listless, clingy?

Many of the above signs are only recognised by professionals used to working with children. If the examining doctor is not aware of the signs of neglect, the nurse caring for the child and his family should make her concerns known.

Emotionally deprived children may be recognised in A&E by their behaviour, which varies from apathetic and depressed to attention-seeking and over-friendly to destructive and aggressive. Questions should be asked as to 'why?', if children's behaviour is clearly abnormal.

Sexually abused children may present in many ways to the A&E department. Clearly, if a child tells of his abuse, the clinical task is much more straightforward than if abnormal physical signs are found incidentally. This is particularly true in young children who have limited language, developmentally delayed children and in any child who is not ready to tell by virtue of fear or coercion.

Examples of presentation are:

- a child may disclose to her mother, the parents want an immediate opinion and come directly to the A&E department
- a seven-year-old girl may be found to be bleeding from the genital area, from an unexplained injury after grandfather who was baby-sitting has left
- a boy of ten years complains of a 'sore bottom' and his mother finds blood on his pants, when there is no history of constipation
- a five-year-old girl has a vaginal discharge and unexplained bruise on her abdomen, grip marks round her thighs and knees
- a twelve-year-old girl is readmitted yet again with 'non-specific abdominal pain'. What is the cause of the stress?
- a fourteen-year-old girl has slashed her arms and taken her second overdose of Paracetamol. Why?
- a thirteen-year-old boy has been found unconscious, he is known to abuse solvents, but has recently run away from home for the fourth time
- a fifteen-year-old girl is brought in overbreathing, the police having been called when she threatened to jump off the top of a block of maisonettes
- a fourteen-year-old girl gives birth to a premature baby in the department, the father not being known.

The physical examination in the possibly sexually abused child may be entirely normal, demonstrate signs consistent with child sexual abuse or confirm child sexual abuse. There are few of the latter signs but gonorrhoea, pregnancy or evidence of semen in the child's vagina clearly confirms child sexual abuse. A laceration or scar of the hymen, attenuation of the hymen with loss of hymenal tissue and laceration or scar of the anal mucosa extending beyond the anal verge on to the perianal skin are highly correlated with child sexual abuse (Royal College of Physicians, 1991). There are also signs such as reflex anal dilatation, anal laxity, and dilated perianal veins which are associated with anal abuse. Other signs such as reddening, that is inflammation perianally or vulvitis, are non-specific and, although they may be 'consistent with' a history of rubbing, are not proof of abuse.

How nursing staff may help abused children and the management of possible abuse

A trained nurse may help make the child's visit to the A&E into a positive one by the way she handles him and his family. Abusing families may be very difficult, but a sympathetic approach to the adults and a calm, firm approach to the child will often defuse a potentially difficult situation. Children usually respond quickly to a caring adult and particularly one who will get down on the floor and play. This is a skilled task and the nurse's observations on the child's behaviour should be recorded.

While the child is weighed, measured or examined, the nurse should

- talk to the child gently
- reassure
- explain what is happening
- explain why, for example, a urine specimen is needed.

When older children are examined a chaperon may be needed, and again the nurse may give comfort and confidence to the child whilst ensuring the child has maximum privacy.

These activities are not to be undervalued — it takes experience and training to handle these sensitive clinical situations well. Other nurses in the A&E department may have more direct responsibility for child protection issues. A liaison health visitor in the department may

- be present to advise, teach and support colleagues dealing with children who may have been abused
- liaise with the family's health visitor
- review 'problematical cases', e.g. unexplained fracture or injury
- review children who are frequent A&E attenders
- audit management within A&E

Difficulties may arise in the A&E department when the nursing staff are concerned about possible child maltreatment and the medical staff are dismissive. In these cases the nurse should talk to senior colleagues and voice the concerns at the time. Subsequently the difficulty should be raised at the regular staff/audit meeting — but with every case the concerns and actions should be clearly recorded and information passed on appropriately.

Out of all the many children seen in A&E each day the few abused children must be recognised, protected and their families helped.

A clinical decision has to be made as to whether to refer a child and his family to social services and the police. Clearly, a balance is necessary, children must be protected but the investigation itself may be traumatic to the family. To help make a reasoned decision more information needs to be collected by

- talking to the child's health visitor
- talking to the child's general practitioner
- obtaining any other third party information
- finding out if the child or family is known to social services
- checking if the child's name is on the child protection register.

It varies as to who in the department collects all this information. A liaison health visitor and a social worker based in the A&E department may undertake some of this work and are invaluable.

It also varies from case to case when the information should be collected. If the child is unconscious, bruised and battered the child is clearly to stay in hospital and the child's clinical care comes first. In such a clear-cut case, however, there are concerns which must be addressed quickly, such as 'Are there other children in the family?' Once the immediate clinical crisis is over, social services should be contacted.

Whether it is safe to let a child go home is a much more difficult question to answer. For example, a child of four years old has been brought to A&E by ambulance following a '999 call' after he has fallen off his bike and broken his arm, the casualty Officer notes he has old, severe bruising of his ear and an injury which looks like a hand slap across his face. In this circumstance further information is needed before the child may go home. In practice a social worker should make this decision. It is not a simple medical decision: he does not require medical admission but the earlier injuries must be investigated and a decision made on the wider issues. This does not mean a hospital admission but it may mean alternative care.

An outline of the management of another case is shown in the Figure 7.1.

Child protection involves a good working relationship between health, the police and social services. These relationships are difficult to maintain and work best if the various professionals meet and work together regularly. Most health districts now have designated (named) nurses, midwives and doctors who are responsible for this work. Increasingly, consultant community paediatricians are being appointed with a particular interest in child maltreatment and will co-ordinate the services. However, it is the nurse and doctor in the clinic who have the most difficult task and they need training and support, both of which may be inadequate.

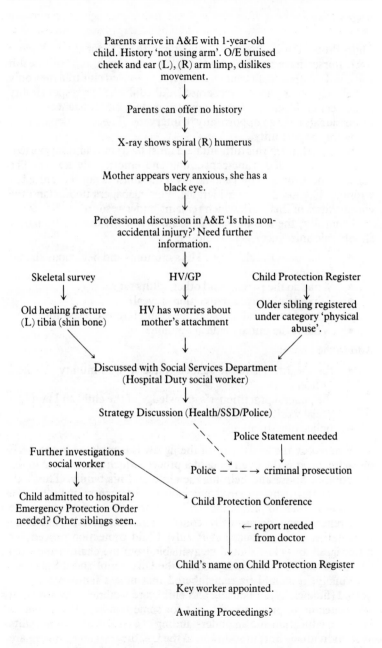

Figure 7.1   Management of Possible Abuse in A&E Department

Summary

Child Protection is a major social issue in the UK for the 1990s and
A&E nurses have an important contribution to make. Child health
and child maltreatment cannot co-exist, but abused children may only
be helped if their plight is recognised. All adults have a responsibility
to protect children, but there are also certain circumstances where
professionals have an opportunity to intervene. The A&E department
offers this opportunity.

Staff working in this difficult field must be trained and supported.
The work is skilled, time-consuming and emotionally taxing. The
consequences for the child and family if the abuse is not recognised or
wrongly diagnosed are considerable. Few managers understand the
complexities of this work which remains under-resourced.

Clinically, the acceptance of the notion of the diagnostic jigsaw
should minimise incorrect diagnoses:

- What does the child say? His symptoms and behaviour should
  be considered.
- What do the parents and other adults say?
- What do physical examinations reveal?
- What do medical investigations (and forensic tests) add?
- What is the initial medical opinion?

Add to the above:

- the health visitor's, school nurse's, Community Medical
  Officers view
- the general practitioner's knowledge of the child and family
- social work assessment
- police investigations.

While only the initial part of the jigsaw is completed in the A&E
department, it is the beginning of a process which should lead to the
cessation of abuse and help for the child and his family. The A&E
staff, in preparing reports and police statements, may have a
continuing role in attending child protection conferences (case
conferences) and occasionally courts. This latter task should be
undertaken by experienced staff only. Child protection procedures
differ in all areas but should be available from the chair of the Area
Child Protection Committee, usually the Director of Social Services.

Finally, it should be remembered that unless families are supported (financially, in housing and child care facilities) child-rearing
will continue to prove too difficult for some families. Prevention is
based on education and an understanding of a child's needs and rights
as an individual. But, in addition, in the UK the least able families are
expected to function well under the greatest stress, especially poverty.

Society must address childhood poverty to improve the chances of impoverished families functioning more adequately. Child sexual abuse would not occur if the child's rights were respected. However, protection of children from sexual abuse is a long way off. Nursing and other professionals can and should respond to child abuse and initiate protective action, but unless the broader structural causes of child abuse and neglect are addressed child abuse will persist.

References

Butler-Sloss, E. (1988) *Report of the Inquiry into Child Abuse in Cleveland 1987*. London: HMSO. pp. 243, 246.

Creighton, S. J. and Noyes, P. (1989) *Child Abuse Trends in England and Wales 1983–87*. London: National Society for the Prevention of Cruelty to Children.

Department of Health (1991a) *Children and Young Persons on Child Protection Registers Year Ending 31 March 1990 in England*. London: Department of Health.

Department of Health (1991b) *Working Together under the Children Act 1989*. London: HMSO.

Hobbs, C. J. (1984) Skull fracture and diagnosis of abuse. *Archives of Disease in Childhood*, 59, p. 246.

Hobbs, C. J. (1986) When are burns non-accidental? *Archives of Disease in Childhood*, 61, p. 357.

Kempe, H. et al. (1962) The battered child syndrome. *Journal of the American Medical Association*, 181, pp. 17–22.

Newell, P. (1989) *Children are People Too: The Case Against Physical Punishment*. London: Bedford Square.

Newlands, M. and Emery, J. S. (1991) Child abuse and cot death. *Child Abuse and Neglect*, 15, pp. 275–8.

Newson, J., and Newson, E. (1965) *Infant Care in an Urban Community*. London: Allen and Unwin.

Robertson, D. N., Barbor, P. and Hull, D. (1982) Unusual injury?: recent injury in normal children and children with suspected non-accidental injury. *British Medical Journal*, 285, p. 1299.

Royal College of Physicians (1991) *Physical Signs of Sexual Abuse in Children: A Report*. London: Royal College of Physicians.

Taitz, L. S. (1988) Child abuse and Osteogenesis Imperfecta. *British Medical Journal*, 296, p. 292.

Wheeler, D. M. and Hobbs, C. J. (1988) Mistakes in the diagnosis of non-accidental injury: 10 years experience. *British Medical Journal*, 296, p. 1233.

Worlock et al. (1986) Patterns of fractures in accidental and non-accidental injury in children: a comparative study. *British Medical Journal*, 292, p. 100.

8 'Protecting' children and 'preventing' child abuse: a consensus or conflict?

Jim Waters

Health visitors are involved in a range of activities which span a continuum from prevention to protection. They are expected to undertake long-term preventive work which involves building up close relationships with families, and also to take quick decisive child protection measures. The polarities of prevention and protection may be felt in daily practice. Health visitors need to develop strategies to resolve the seemingly contradictory position in which they find themselves and to build their confidence.

This chapter is based on the author's experience of a joint agencies project in Warrington which, between August 1988 and January 1991, saw a specialist health visitor attached to an NSPCC protection team. Each child protection team comprised social workers engaged exclusively in protective work. The chapter considers the origins of the prevention–protection dichotomy, looks at the resulting pressures on health visitors, and offers possible solutions.

The paradigms of 'protection' and 'prevention'

Sadly, the 'child abuse industry' has been one of the major growth concerns of the late twentieth century. The pioneering work in the

1960s of Henry Kempe and his associates discovered the 'battered baby syndrome', and since that time the work of protecting children has had many name changes (Calder and Waters, 1991). Different types of abuse have been discovered, most recently, for example, network abuse. There has been a number of public enquiries and a good deal of public pressure and outrage. There has been intensive growth in legal changes and policy statements from government departments. Many public, government and other concerns have focused on the fact that different professionals are required to 'work together' better.

One of the responses to the public demand to get child abuse work right has been for professionals to tend towards specialising. Hence, 'child protection work' has become an entity. Indeed, dedicated 'teams' have been established which specialise totally in child protection work. The tendency seems to have been to give an investigative and assessment brief to these teams rather than a healing or treatment focus.

In contrast, 'preventive child care work' has not developed as an entity since its inception in the late sixties and early seventies. While the very term 'prevention' has a lot of associations and connotations for operational practitioners, it is likely to be less clear and to include a more global notion of what work it actually involves than the concept of 'child protection'. In particular, the boundaries and indeed punctuation points between the tasks of investigation, assessment, 'treatment' and 'healing' are less clear.

One way of looking at these forms of work — 'preventive' work and 'protection' work — could be to see them as 'paradigms'. A paradigm is a set of beliefs, understandings and concepts which organise expectations and behaviours over time. They are a form of archetype or master copy of belief or understanding. The paradigms become set or established and can become quite difficult to change. They are a clustering of beliefs rather than a set programme. The beliefs are more likely to be covert rather than overt. The beliefs are more likely to be implicit rather than explicit. The usefulness of a paradigm is that it allows a number of people to stand behind those beliefs and to be committed to them (Kahn, 1970).

Figure 8.1 crystallises the 'paradigms' of 'Child Protection' and 'Prevention of Child Abuse' which workers encounter in regular practice on each working day. They also make sense to the health visitors and social workers who have spoken to us about their practice. I make no apologies for the fact that the characters appear like heroes from Bunyan's *Pilgrim's Progress*, rather than embodying the princi-ples and characteristics underlining a notion of 'respect for person', with which we are inculcated in training. Rather, the statements that the characters make in Figure 8.1 are stereotypical responses. We feel

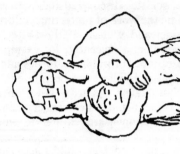

I am Child Protection.

I always protect the child.

I will give tough messages to families about the care of their children.

I ensure that parents know that they are responsible for their children.

I will work with a legal mandate.

If you don't clean this house up . . . I will come down on you like a ton of bricks.

This family impairs the development of these children.

I just have to get things straight with this family.

I'll tell the case conference what the family needs.

If this family doesn't change it's their fault.

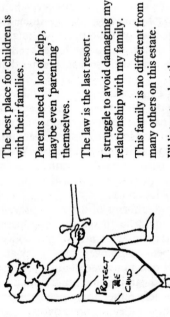

I am Prevention.

I struggle to ensure the children do not go into care.

The best place for children is with their families.

Parents need a lot of help, maybe even 'parenting' themselves.

The law is the last resort.

I struggle to avoid damaging my relationship with my family.

This family is no different from many others on this estate.

I'll listen to what the case conference attenders have to say.

If this family doesn't change it's my fault.

Figure 8.1 Paradigmatic 'Child Protection' and 'Prevention of Child Abuse' Responses

that they are ideal typical responses to ethical dilemmas presented by the work context within which health visitors find themselves. It is also possible to extend this stereotype by seeing a 'masculine/ feminine' polarity: the masculine, comprising 'control' and the strength of child protection, versus the feminine, comprising the 'nurture' response of child abuse prevention.

These polarities are not newly discovered. In an article in 1989, Taylor and Tilley recognised that health visitors were tending to go 'underground' in an 'undercover operation' to resolve the control responsibilities of their role in child protection work. These authors said that this especially occurred when the health visitors were having to shift their footing with families of children under five, about whom concerns were raised by other professionals or about whom concerns became crystallised around a notion of child protection.

It is suggested that health visitors struggle to make sense of their work with families in the context of this ethical dilemma. The main focus, of course, is on the process of trying to get families to change or to agree to change or to want to change for the betterment, improvement and care of their children.

Health visitor's caseload — challenges and dilemmas

In response to this task, health visitors are continually up against the question: Are they agents of social control, or are they agents in the service of a health promotion, educative programme, active agents in the promotion of nurture? The point at which health visitors seem to feel most anxious is when they have a sense that they are working in a vacuum left by other professionals, or when there is growing concern that a child or children are in danger but they fear a referral to a 'child protection' service might either get an over-reaction or no response at all.

Figure 8.2 shows families on a health visitor's case load. It represents families for whom a health visitor is responsible. Circle One represents children on the child protection register. Circle Two represents children not on the register but about whom there are continuing or growing concerns. Circle Three represents children in families where there are no concerns as yet or at least the concerns have not yet become focused.

In terms of the 'polarities', children in Circle Three do not present a problem. The health visitor's role in the screening of health care for the under-fives, immunisation and the like can seem to work like clockwork (although I am not suggesting that this is universally true), and management problems here are about the numbers involved. In the main though, most families are good clinic attenders and want to provide the best health care possible for their children.

Children in Circle One might, in many senses, be expected to present the major difficulties. After all, these are the children who are identified as at risk or who have been abused or who are presented as the greatest 'potential risk'. There will be an identified keyworker — a social worker who is the co-ordinator for the case. The problems here seem to be about maintaining contact levels at agreed rates and as agreed in the child protection plan. It may be that the health visitor cannot complete all the required tasks, and there may be issues about contact and relationships with the family — dealing with an angry family, for example. In a sense, however, the role is fairly clear.

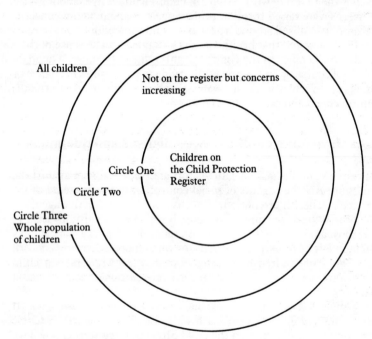

Figure 8.2   Families on a Health Visitor's Caseload

By contrast, children in Circle Two seem to present the greatest difficulties to health visitors. The 'identification' and 'definition' of risk is much more shadowy. Here, health visitors would be in the frontline position. They would perhaps be the first to identify the problem, for example a family who were emotionally abusing their children or where hygiene or home conditions were seriously risky. They would have to see this family whilst maintaining on-going responsibility for a large number of other families.

Having identified these 'at risk' families, and assuming they have discussed and shared concerns with their managers, health visitors would usually identify that their greatest challenges would then be with other professionals and agencies to get them to accept their (i.e. the health visitor's) definition or assessment of these families as 'at risk' or 'in need' of services. Access to resources for children in Circle Two is usually held by other professional agencies. Notable among these would be the social services department, which overwhelmingly controls most of the resources needed: nurseries, family centres, playgroups, home care and family support. Often the health visitor's assessment is no guarantee of matching a resource to a need. Other agencies or professionals will often operate a 'gatekeeping' response. Their task would be to 'gatekeep' a very scarce resource, and they would therefore wish to complete another assessment. This is usually seen by health visitors as being conducted in order to provide good reasons why the resources are not provided. The sense is therefore of 'playing a game' with undeniably scarce resources. This is a game which leaves the health visitor feeling that their assessment is devalued or at best undervalued.

Children in Circle Two are between child 'protection' and 'prevention' of child abuse. This is the true interface between these two areas of work. Among the children with whom health visitors would be concerned in this category are children who have been de-registered. The whole responsibility for visiting and monitoring the children in these families is felt to have fallen entirely to the health visitor. Other types of case which the health visitor feels she or he has been left to handle are those of children who have not been subject to a child protection case conference, but about whom health visitors and other professionals remain highly concerned. An example might be where nursery and health visitors are continuing to be concerned about a family for whom a service is not being provided by other agencies.

Another issue or dilemma is whether or not to 'invoke' child protection procedures. This may feel like a huge step to health visitors. Once families are referred to a 'child protection team', there is a sense that a new dynamic takes over: the professional response moves into a crisis or investigative dynamic. The mode is therefore one of urgent crisis. In terms of the paradigms, the 'child protection worker' becomes operational and the 'prevention' role disappears. Often the punctuation between these two tasks is not clear to the family and may not be made clear either to the health visitor. Nevertheless, a new urgency about 'safe' or 'not safe' appears. Controlling the family in order to ensure the safety of the children becomes or seems to become the priority task.

To summarise so far, health visitors find themselves working in a grey area, and when they identify a 'need' they will often have their assessment replicated by another agency. When a child is 'at risk', the health visitor has to make a decision. Often the decision will be based on a notion of the paradigms of child protection and child abuse prevention. The dilemma may seem quite a difficult one for health visitors: their sense may be one of deciding whether to either mobilise a crisis investigation or to continue to carry the case.

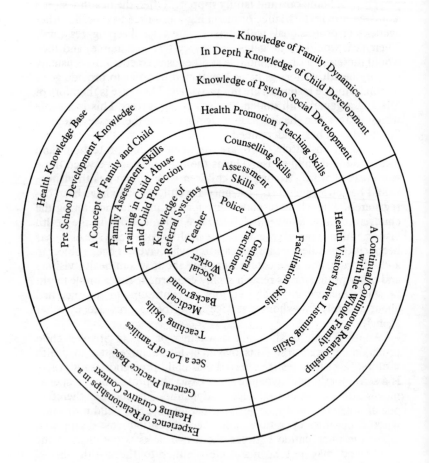

Figure 8.3   A Skills Wheel: What Health Visitors said they could add to the skills of other professionals

The skills contribution of the health visitor

A sample of over thirty health visitors were asked how confident, on a scale of 0–10, they felt themselves to be in the area of child protection. Approximately 70 per cent declared themselves to be feeling unconfident. Despite this, when we analyzed the skills of health visitors, we found they possessed an impressive array of skills, talents and experience. We asked over thirty health visitors/community nurses to add their skills to those of particular professional colleagues. The result, in relation to four closely allied professionals, is shown in Figure 8.3, the 'Skills Wheel'. This demonstrates that often, by virtue of their training in an established and highly creditable area of practice, which is usually longer than that of most other professionals who may be sitting around the child protection case conference table, they have considerable skills and insights to offer.

Most health visitors will, for instance, have gained a recognised nursing qualification and will have exercised this qualification through some kind of management responsibility, such as running a hospital ward as a ward sister, or in some supervisory role in the community. Also, unlike other professionals, excluding class teachers, they will see a huge range of children — indeed, virtually all the under-fives. They will therefore have a basis for comparison between children who are subject to child protection concerns and those who are not.

These points do not need emphasising for health visitors, and other chapters in this book have explored the important issue of the health visitor's skills, training and experience in relation to confidence, security and self-esteem. But these points do need to be made to other professionals. The skills wheel, completed in a workshop setting, yielded for our health visitors group some surprising insights. The skills wheel could perhaps be one way of helping health visitors challenge their lack of confidence about their skills in assessment and what they can offer.

Where health visitors may feel themselves particularly disadvantaged, in comparison with other professionals working at the interface between child protection and child prevention work, is the area of 'team work'. Effective teams are about meeting each other's people's 'needs' and supporting and helping colleagues. Many other professionals have been organised into teams over a longer period than health visitors.

The traditional model for health visiting is for the health visitor to see a large number of families alone, rarely undertaking joint visits. The health visitor in this model operates mainly as a 'one person band', keeping their own notes, doing their own thing. The model for emulation here, of course, is the family practitioner. Often a number of health visitors may be based in a clinic which is part of a building containing a number of GPs working together in a joint practice. The health visitor in this model reports back to a manager or senior nurse who will then discuss cases and share concerns.

The Warrington project and team work

One model of health visitor attachment, as existed in Warrington, comprises a health visitor specifically associated with a child protection project, team or scheme. Alternative models to this, but with a less close attachment, may be liaison posts or an officer with special responsibility for child protection.

There are many advantages and some disadvantages to the attachment model. One major issue is whether the health visitor becomes 'colonised' or feels she or he is becoming inducted into a different operational practice discipline. Another major dilemma is how the crossover management between the different disciplines is arranged. An issue for the attached health visitors in Warrington was their relationship with the 'generic' health visitors who had a more traditional role. The specialist attached health visitors would also have to confront many problems about where they saw themselves in relation to control dilemmas (i.e. would they see themselves as being part of a child protection investigation, for example?). What was their 'health' as opposed to their 'social' role in relation to the familes with whom they worked?

The experience in Warrington of health visitor attachments to child protection teams was on the whole a positive one. The two health visitors demonstrated over time a huge level of experience and skills as a result of their attachment. Because they were part of a social work team with an investigative brief, they were clearly able to communicate their knowledge of this process to their colleagues. They also became regular court and case conference attenders, areas of work in which generic health visitors would recognise that they have not had much opportunity to develop and increase skills. The specialists therefore came to develop an array of skills and competencies which they were well able to share with their wider agency health visitor colleagues.

The team concept seems crucial. It is therefore important to consider practical ways in which health visitors might take forward their work concerns in order to create the most supportive environment possible for themselves and their practice. A practical model is offered here, but it is recognised that not all health visitors will be able or willing to set up teams. Are the health visitors available to be a team? Do they want to be a team? Are they available to each other for discussion of work and exposure of each other's work and cases?

The traditional model of health visiting practice does not lend itself easily to a notion of operating as a team. If the health visitor has to visit a large number of homes (primary and secondary visits), a discussion forum with other peers, or indeed even with managers, may often be seen as an encumbrance or an unnecessary interference with the identified job in hand. It may seem that there is just simply not the time to do it. There are a lot of possibilities for health visitors working in groups. Working as a 'team' is only one possible option.

Coaching, consultation, live supervision, and management

Another possibility may be for health visitors to offer 'coaching' for each other. Coaching is about 'support' and 'advice'. It is not about gossip. It is about focused and clear listening to each other through sharing cases, hypothesising about cases, and sharing ideas and solutions. The 'coach' would need to be clearly aware of being a possible candidate for coaching both in the giving and receiving of coaching, and would also need to be clear about what exactly was being asked for in the coaching relationship.

Offering consultation to practice is another form of coaching, but with a more focused and formalised task set for it. The consultant would be another health visitor colleague, who would need to work at being neutral or 'multi-positional'. It was found that the specialist attached health visitors in Warrington were often providing consultation to their colleagues. The fact that the health visitors were attached to a child protection team gave them a high degree of credibility in the performance of this role of consultant to co-colleagues. The fact that they were 'peers', rather than managers, was valuable in the sense that areas of performance could be more safely opened up. Risks were therefore felt to be less.

In some instances, and again where there is some real control exercised on size of case load, it may be possible for health visitors to offer each other 'live consultation'. Live consultation is observation of an interaction or an encounter either within the same room or from behind a one-way screen or via a video monitor. Although this practice is usually best achieved where there are one-way screens available and, if possible, video tape replay facilities, it may be possible in some instances for the live consultant to accompany a health visitor on a visit or to sit in during a clinic interview. The advantage of live consultation, sometimes referred to as live supervision, is that the consultant gets a real feel of the interaction between the client and health visitor and can offer on-the-spot guidance and advice which may be of very real benefit and help to both the patient or family and the health visitor concerned.

The aim of any consultation forum is to be as useful as possible. The key is not to be 'right' or to not be 'wrong', but to be as 'helpful' or as facilitative as possible. Coaching and consultation are not about problem-solving but about giving information, stating and opening up possibilities, rather than closing down options in a search for linear solutions.

Live consultation is perhaps more familiar to social work and, indeed, family therapy practice, where it is often used as a part of the work with families. In the Dangerous Families Assessment described by the Rochdale NSPCC Special Unit Team, live consultation was very much a part of the process of assessment of families where the major issue was the assessment of dangerous familes (Dale et al., 1986).

What is being suggested here is that a live consultation process may be a one-off service offered to health visitors who perhaps want to learn and increase their skills and make changes and interventions in families which are helpful to the clients or patients.

Supervision, or management consultation, is where an account-able or responsible manager directly supervises the work of a health visitor. Again, in terms of the traditional health visitor, this is provided by a nurse manager. A major problem in the context of health visiting is that the nursing officer has such extensive areas of responsibility, and the health visitors themselves see such a large number of families, that the amount of time available for discussing families where there are concerns is exceedingly limited. As changes in health authorities take place, the pressure on management time for health visitors is likely to increase rather than decrease. Management availability for health visiting staff is likely to reduce over the next few years. This raises the need for an urgent consideration of alternatives as a supplement or as a complement to traditional management structures for health visiting.

What is therefore being suggested here is that there may perhaps be a continuum which health visitors ought to seriously consider when they are thinking about cases and about what they need to ask for in terms of support or help in making assessments or interventions with families. It is perhaps particularly important to get this help or service when health visitors are looking at the children who are caught between the polarities of 'child protection' and 'child abuse preven-tion' work. Having considered the continuum from informal case discussion, through coaching and consultation, to formal supervision and management, the health visitors would need to decide which of these approaches might best be used to shift or move on an interview or an observation of a family. They may then consider what exactly they would want from the process of the intervention.

Table 8.1 seeks to demonstrate the difference between coaching, consultation, live supervision, and management. This comprises a series of questions with different emphases.

Table 8.1   Methods of supporting health visitors

Coaching	Consultation	Live Supervision	Management
Questions for the 'coach' to ask in relation to 'family'	Questions for the consultant to ask in relation to the family	Questions the consultant may ask	Questions the management may wish to ask
1. Is this a 'family' who keeps *things* the same?	1. What three key processes in this family maintain things as they are?	1. What three key beliefs are there *right now* in this family?	1. What three key actions do you need to make and in what time scale?
2. What would be the 'cheekiest' question that could be asked about this 'family'?	2. What three questions dare you not ask in relation to this family and risk?	2. How do the family/ family members organise each other and the health visitor? (suggest 3 ways)	2. What support systems are available from your peers/ colleagues to enable (1) above to take place?
3. What *three* major concerns are there in this family and how are they connected?	3. In what three major ways do the family attempt to 'organise' the health visitor?	3. What is 'unsaid' and what would the health visitor be most afraid of saying/ declaring or asking?	3. In what way do you want me to manage? (How) and How will we review the usefulness of this process?
4. What would be the most radical suggestion that could be made with regard to this family?	4. If you were to look back, at a point in the future, how would you like this family to look?	4. What would be the most useful and positive intervention or 'ritual' that could be made? (check if this is accepted by the colleague?)	4. What is your 'cheekiest' thought about my management of you?

There are a number of similar points that have to be borne in mind when health visitors agree to engage in this process: *the ground rules* should be agreed with the consultee. Ground rules for the consultant include:

- Only offer or give help if you are clearly asked. If you are asked, check out your mandate. Are you being asked to be a coach, consultant or manager?
- Raise questions rather than make statements.

- Do not become too easily drawn into problem-solving. Usually our colleagues are very good at problem-solving; they would benefit instead from imaginative or creative methods of developing information or insights rather than action points. Instead of quick answers, suggest and look for 'possibilities'.
- When coaching, avoid being critical. Notice when your colleagues take things 'personally', comment on this, and think about how you can avoid being caught in a 'critical frame'.
- Look for the 'paradigms'. Try to see if there are 'child protection' and 'child abuse prevention' polarities in the beliefs. Notice how possibilities can exist between the polarities.

Seeking to resolve the conflicts

Health visitors possess a range of skills and competencies which can contribute to the protection of children. Often these skills are not properly exercised because the emphasis in their work is seemingly on preventive care. Such shifts in approach can be uncomfortable and threatening, and as a result, quite understandably, health visitors may pull back and avoid protective action.

The conflicts inherent in the health visitor's role may in part be overcome by first openly acknowledging the contradictions and then by seeking to address them. This involves understanding the skills and capabilities which health visitors bring to the protective task.

It is not simply a case of health visitors recognising their contribution, but equally importantly that other professionals do so too, and that methods are then developed of supporting health visitors in this work. This chapter has discussed some approaches which may be taken.

In seeking to operationalise these models, it should be understood that there are powerful forces which may militate against their implementation — not least resources, management structures and the prevailing paradigm. The Warrington experience has shown, however, that the conflicts can be broken down and, in so doing, children are offered greater protection and the professional community enriched.

References

Calder, M. and Waters, J. (1991) Child protection: what's in a name? Presentation at BASPCAN, Leicester.
Dale, P., Davies, M., Morrison, T. and Waters, J. (1986) *Dangerous Families? A Systematic Model of Assessment of Child Abuse Families*. London: Tavistock.

Kahn, T. S. (1970) *The Structure of Scientific Revolutions*, 2nd edn. Chicago: University of Chicago Press.
Taylor, S. and Tilley N. (1989) Health visitors and child protection: conflict, contradictions and ethical dilemmas. *Health Visitor*, 62, (9), pp. 273–275.

Acknowledgements

The author wishes to thank Jean Carter and Margaret O'Sullivan, Specialist Child Protection Health Visitors, Warrington Health Authority, and also Elaine Fiveash, Special Health Visitor, Rochdale.

9 Putting it all together: the Children Act 1989

Wendy Stainton Rogers and Jeremy Roche

The Lord Chancellor heralded the Children Act as 'the most comprehensive and far reaching reform of child care law which has come before Parliament in living memory'. This chapter is intended to do three things in relation to this new legislation. First, it sets out to give some sense of why this legislation was needed. What is it seeking to do, and what problems is it designed to overcome? Secondly, the chapter will summarise the main legal changes the Act will bring about, particularly in relation to child protection. In what ways does it seek to protect children from harm in innovative and better ways? And thirdly, it will seek to explore some of the Act's main implications for health visitors and nurses, both in terms of their day-to-day practice, and more especially in terms of their contribution to keeping children safe and helping to prevent them being mistreated. In other words, in what ways does the Act offer health visitors and nurses new and better ways of working with children and families? In this chapter a broad definition of 'child protection' is adopted, which regards, as indeed does the Act itself, preventive work as critically important and always preferable to crisis intervention. Keeping children safe and making sure they have the opportunities they need for healthy and happy development has far more to do with avoiding them being abused or neglected in the first place, than it has to do with intervening once the harm has been done.

The Children Act received royal assent in November 1989 and was implemented in October 1991. It arose out of two separate sets of deliberations about the inadequacies of the then current law in relation to children. First, in 1985 the Social Services Select Committee published a *Review of Child Care Law*, which examined a number of shortcomings in public law, specifically the legislative basis of statutory intervention such as child protection and care proceedings. Secondly, in 1988 the Law Commission produced a *Review of Child Care Law: Guardianship and Custody*, which examined problems to do with private law, specifically disputes between private individuals such as over who should have custody of children following divorce. Not only were both areas of law seen to be overcomplex and unable to properly address children's needs, it was felt that the divisions between them were unhelpful. Further fuel was added to the debate by a number of public inquiry reports, including those on the deaths of Jasmine Beckford and Kimberley Carlile and also the Cleveland Report, which together raised a number of issues concerning the balance between the need to intervene in families and the need to avoid subjecting children and families to practices which, in themselves, were abusive.

However, the major reasons for change were probably a number of fundamental shifts in attitude. These had to do in particular with the way children are perceived. In the past they were treated very much as their parents' property, and there was a widespread conviction that parents had an inalienable right to bring their children up as they chose. This view had become increasingly challenged within a system of welfare which acknowledged a child's right to protection from cruelty and neglect. However, more recently still, there have been growing concerns that the outcome of interventionist strategies for children was that parental power was simply taken over by professional power. This resulted, in Butler-Sloss's memorable phrase, in children becoming treated as the 'objects of professional concern' rather than people in their own right — with wishes and feelings of their own, a right to be told what was happening and why, and a growing ability, as they matured, to make decisions for themselves. The Gillick appeal ruling in 1986 was a turning point in this regard, as it identified in law that once young people gain sufficient intelligence and understanding to understand the consequences of particular decisions, for example the use of contraception, professionals should respect this capability and begin to treat them as agents in their own right.

A second, parallel, change in perception had to do with shifts in our understanding, more generally, of disability. Largely in response to the way people with disabilities have lobbied for being treated as people first and foremost, who happen to have a disability, rather than

being stigmatised as 'the disabled', it became increasingly acknowledged that when this principle is applied to children, their needs and
rights needed to be met primarily as children, entitled to the same life-
chances as other children and to the same sorts of childhood,
particularly growing up in their own families wherever possible. This
viewpoint had very considerable implications within the drafting of
the Children Act, since it demands that services for children with
disabilities must first be channelled, wherever possible, through their
families; and second, they must be determined by the child's needs,
not by the bureaucratic constraints of service-providers.

Finally, the Act responds to a fundamental change in perception
of the importance to a child of their links with their family, including
their wider family, and their community, including the child's
religious, racial, cultural and linguistic roots. There has been a
growing recognition that children do not just need the physical basis
of a nurturing upbringing, such as adequate hygiene, nutrition and
opportunities for play. As importantly, their growing sense of identity
and their future capacities for satisfying and supportive social
relationships mean that, unless they maintain close links with their
parents, siblings and people who are significant to them, including
their wider family, they can all too easily be set adrift. Children cut off
from their families and communities then have to struggle in the
world, very much alone and lacking the networks of support on which
we all depend. The Act therefore seeks to reinforce rather than
undermine these links, and to ensure that whenever and wherever
children are looked after — in day and residential care and all other
services provided to them — these services are appropriate in terms of
the child's culture, race, religion, racial origins and linguistic
background.

Consequently, the Act is a massive piece of legislation which is
deliberately interconnected. While the temptation may be just to look
for those specific 'bits' which are obviously most salient, this would
miss the most essential point — that the Act is not intended just to
tinker in a minor way with a few specifics, but to bring about a whole
new approach to the way children are cared for, brought up and
looked after in this country, and the services they need provided to
them. In consequence, for anybody to respond by merely seeking to
achieve 'old solutions' with 'new measures' would be to miss out on
the enormous potential of the Act to change things fundamentally for
the better — with children's lives, wellbeing and futures the
beneficiaries. This is not to say that everything will be easy, or that
there are not massive problems to be overcome to do with severe
resource constraints, bureaucratic inertia, professional jealousies,
and, indeed, genuine conflicts of interest. But unusually, this
legislation, despite its critics and its undoubted shortcomings, has

been widely applauded across political and professional divides.
While its practical implications are certainly challenging, its intentions are seen to be extremely worthwhile.

The changes the Act is seeking to achieve

There are five main areas in which changes are being brought about.
These are: changes in the legal system itself; a new model for
parenthood; changes in service provision; specific changes in child
protection; and changes in the provision of substitute care. Each of
these will be covered briefly, in turn. If, having read these sections,
you wish to know more, you should consult *The Children Act 1989: An
Introductory Guide for the NHS* (HMSO). More extensive training is
provided in *The Children Act 1989: Putting it into Practice* (Open
University) or *The Children Act 1989: A Training and Study Guide for
Health Professionals* (HMSO) on which this chapter is partially based.

Changing the legal system

While it has been accepted in law for some time now that, in making
decisions about a child's upbringing and safety, it must be the child's
welfare which is the paramount consideration, the way the law
actually operated militated against this. The adversarial ethos of
proceedings often meant that adults fought against each other to win
in protected fights, which often left children in limbo for months and
even years at critical stages in their development. The outcomes were
frequently not the best ones for the child, because that consideration
got lost in the heat of the battle. The child's welfare was often decided
by who could shout the loudest or bring out the biggest guns, not by a
careful, systematic and dispassionate examination of the child's needs
and circumstances. And all too often children's own wishes were
ignored or not even ascertained. The law clearly needed to be made
more child-centred — designed and run in such a way that children's
needs (and not the court's, the professional's or the lawyer's needs)
determined what happens.

The first part of the Act, therefore, includes three critical,
overarching principles:

- When determining issues concerning the child's upbringing
  or property, the child's welfare is the paramount consideration. A check-list is provided to help such decisions be made
  effectively.
- In making decisions, delay is likely to be harmful to the child,
  and should be avoided.

- The court should not intervene (i.e. make an order) unless doing so is better for the child than making no order at all.

The check-list was introduced to ensure that courts at all levels and all over the country took into account a wider range of issues about children's circumstances, including their physical, emotional and educational needs, the effects upon them of any change in circumstances, their age, sex and background and other characteristics such as their racial origin or any special needs they may have. It also covers looking at possible harm children may suffer and the capability of each of their parents and others to meet their needs. The check-list, in addition, directs the court to consider the range of orders they can make — in other words, it allows for a different order to be made than the one applied for, if this would be better for the child. In particular, this may mean that instead, say, of making a care order, the court might decide to make a residence order placing the child under supervision (the criteria of 'significant harm' would have to be satisfied here). The check-list applies to contested proceedings following parental divorce or separation — for example, where there is a dispute about where the child will live — and in care and supervision proceedings. It does not apply to cases involving emergency protection, including assessment during an investigation, where ensuring the safety of the child takes precedence over these wider issues.

The Act also completely revises the relationships between courts and introduces, at magistrate's court level, a new court altogether. This, the Family Proceedings Court, brings together the previous juvenile and domestic court functions in relation to children's upbringing, so that, with a number of small exceptions, one court makes decisions about children's welfare — whether following divorce, in care proceedings, or to resolve disputes about specific issues, for example whether or not a child should receive medical treatment to which the child's parents refuse consent. The three-tier system of courts remains, with proceedings also able to be heard in the County and High Courts. However, these now have 'concurrent jurisdiction', which means that with minor exceptions the same rules apply, the courts have the same powers, and cases can thus be transferred from one to another as appropriate. Thus, while it is expected that the majority of cases will at least start in the local magistrate's court, those that are particularly difficult, in legal terms, for example where there is complex medical evidence in dispute or foreign legislation is involved, will generally start in or be transferred to a higher court.

This focus on hearing most cases in local magistrates' courts is intended to mean that cases can be dealt with more immediately, more cheaply and more conveniently, as, for example, parents and witnesses will have less travelling to do. It is also hoped that this can lead to a closer partnership between local courts and the agencies and staff working in the area, so that lines of communication are better, problems can be resolved more effectively, and crises tackled speedily and efficiently. In order for this to happen, the magistrates comprising Family Proceedings Courts and court staff have all been specially trained in the Children Act, and, as time progresses, will receive more training, including, it is hoped, more collaborative training with professional and voluntary agencies in the field of child development and child welfare. At the same time, the judiciary has also received specific training on the Act, including, for the first time, training from child care and child welfare professionals, including paediatricians, community physicians and child psychiatrists.

Another major change has to do with the way decisions are to be made. In general terms, courts will work with written reports prepared and made available to the court and parties to the proceedings ahead of time. This is intended to facilitate transfer of cases, to avoid busy professionals needing to attend court, and to work towards a less adversarial system of decision-making. In this regard, courts are expected to become more active in reviewing all the pertinent information and seeking the best outcome for the child, as opposed to merely adjudicating between warring 'sides'.

Finally, and critically, court procedures have been amended to enable them to take seriously the 'no delay' principle. The Act introduces a system of 'preliminary hearings' administered by the Clerk to the Justices, in which a timetable is set for the case (often this will be a matter of weeks) and decisions made on what information the court will require and — crucially — will be prepared to consider. These preliminary hearings will be critical in that, unless a case is made at them for certain information to be required, for example a medical examination of the child, such information cannot be decided upon and included at a later stage, except with the leave of the court. Similarly, the 'no order' principle enshrines another element of the Act's philosophy — that legal sanctions and intervention should be a last resort. Wherever possible, disputes about a child's welfare or future should be sorted out by voluntary arrangements, backed up, where appropriate, by informal written agreements, in partnership with parents. Courts will only be prepared, and indeed empowered, to intervene, once genuine attempts to find a resolution by informal, voluntary means have been made and have failed.

Changing the concept of parenthood

The Act introduces a new term — *parental responsibility*. Its actual definition is not all that different from before, but what is completely new is how it operates and what it implies. First, it lasts throughout a child's minority. Married parents and unmarried mothers have it automatically and can only lose it if the child is adopted or freed for adoption. Otherwise, they retain parental responsibility for their children until they reach eighteen years of age. Others can gain parental responsibility in a variety of ways: unmarried fathers by an agreement with the mother, or by court order; others, such as relatives and foster parents, by a court order. Local authorities can only gain it through the court making a care or emergency protection order, i.e. this is no longer possible via a 'parental rights resolution', which the Act has abolished.

The second important point is that, when somebody other than the child's parent acquires parental responsibility, they do not take it over from the child's parent(s), except in the case of adoption, but share it with them. For example, where a local authority gains parental responsibility when the court makes a care order, the child's parents continue to have parental responsibility, although the local authority may limit how the parents exercise it. It might direct that the child live elsewhere, for instance with relatives, and that their contact with their child should be supervised. However, they would still be expected to participate, alongside the child her/himself, in decisions made about their child, and would be kept informed about the child's whereabouts and circumstances.

This idea of sharing parental responsibility makes redundant the concepts of 'custody' and 'care and control' following divorce. These are now obsolete and have no meaning under current law. Both married parents, whenever the divorce took place, now have parental responsibility. Following the Act, the 'no order' principle means that, from now on, when parents divorce or separate, they are expected to come to an agreement together about arrangements for their children. The law will not intervene unless there is an irresolvable dispute. However, if the disagreement does go to law, the Children Act provides highly specific resolutions to specific issues. It does not award 'parental responsibility' to one or other parent, as both keep it, but, instead, one of four orders (called Section 8 Orders) may be made:

- Residence Order
- Contact Order
- Prohibited Steps Order
- Specific Issues Order

Probably the most important is the *Residence Order*, since this not only determines where the child shall live, but gives certain powers to the person in whose name the order has been made, including parental responsibility if they do not already hold it, for example in the case of an unmarried father. This is one of the routes by which a relative or a foster parent may gain parental responsibility. A *Contact Order* is to resolve disputes about what used to be called 'access' (another redundant term, and contact means considerably more — it includes letters and phone calls). A Section 8 Contact Order only applies to private law. Disputes about contact with children in care are resolved by a Section 34 Contact Order. Divorces which preceded the Act are subject to various transitional arrangements. The main one is that both parents will automatically have parental responsibility for their children, though the fact that a parent now has parental responsibility will not entitle her or him to behave in any way which is incompatible with an existing order, for example by removing the child from the parent who has a custody order.

The *Prohibited Steps Order* and the *Specific Issues Order* are intended to resolve disputes about how parental responsibility is exercised. A Prohibited Steps Order might be sought by a parent wanting to prevent the child receiving cosmetic surgery. A Specific Issues order could be applied for, for example, when parents disagree about the child's education — it could direct which school the child should attend. However, these orders may also be used in other situations, when people other than parents wish to intervene. For example, one could be sought by a hospital to gain permission for a child to have life-saving surgery.

Finally, following divorce, a court may make a Family Assistance Order if the circumstances of the case are exceptional. Its aim is to provide help to families in the immediate aftermath of family division, particularly where there has been a lot of conflict. The order may be used, say, to involve a court welfare officer helping to see that arrangements for maintaining contact are got off to a reasonable start.

Changing the system of service provision

The Act offers a basis for a more effective system of service provision, based upon the real needs of children and their families. Prior to the implementation of the Act, provision had evolved out of a long series of piecemeal legislative and organisational changes, resulting in a lack of co-ordination between the different statutory sectors — social services, health, education, housing — and with the voluntary agencies. The consequence was an unwieldy system in which any individual child's or family's requirements were met — if at all, and often not very effectively — by an imprecise matching of their needs to what happened to be available in the locality, via a muddled patchwork of largely independent and uncoordinated bureaucratic systems. What was seen to be needed was a move to a needs-led system of planning. This was to consist of a systematic audit of the scale and range of services actually required by those children in the area with the most pressing needs, coupled with a review of all services already available. The aim of this process is to create an efficient system in which gaps in provision can be plugged, overlaps avoided, and underused services closed down. In this way it is hoped that scarce resources can be utilised more efficiently and the delivery of services can be tailored to the specific, individual needs of particular children and their families.

However, it is important to acknowledge that the economic and political climate dictated, when the Act was being drafted, that, while some basic fundamentals were to apply to all children, service provision was to be targeted on the most needy. The Act therefore introduces another important new term — 'children in need'. It should not be confused with a child with 'specific educational needs' (SEN) under the 1981 Education Act, since its definition is considerably more comprehensive, encompassing both children with disabilities and those whose health and development will be impaired unless services are provided, i.e. their needs relate to social and economic deprivation. The Act defines a child as disabled if she or he is blind, deaf or dumb, or suffers from mental disorder of any kind or is substantially and permanently handicapped by illness, injury or congenital deformity. This definition mirrors the National Assistance Act 1948, whose somewhat outdated language shows.

The function of the composite definition of 'in need' is to establish those children and families who are entitled to a range of services. This has to do with the difference in law between *powers* (i.e. the discretion to do something), indicated by the term 'may', and *duties* (i.e. the obligation to do something), indicated by the term 'shall'. In general terms, the Act gives local authorities powers to provide services for all children, but places them under a duty to provide services for 'children in need'. While a number of voluntary organisations and some professionals are unhappy about the drawing together of children 'in need' through social and economic deprivation, and children and their families facing the challenges of their disabilities, the intention of the Act is to ensure that children who are disabled are entitled to the services they need, in order to 'minimise the effect . . . of their disabilities' and to 'give such children the chance to lead lives which are as normal as possible'. The idea is that their entitlement to services is as children first and foremost, and to bring these children within the commitment to enable them, as far as possible, to be cared for and brought up by their families.

In order to rationalise service provision, the Act introduces a system of assessment and registration. The purpose of assessment is twofold. First, in the usual way, it is intended to identify each child's (and their family's) strengths and weaknesses and hence their needs for services. In this way, in theory at least, a tailored profile of service provision can be arranged. However, the second purpose is more innovatory and is potentially far-reaching. By identifying all the children 'in need' in their area, and by specifying what needs each of them has, local authorities are expected to gather together the information necessary to plan in conjunction with other agencies — including health authorities — and voluntary organisations and self-help groups, a comprehensive, integrated, effective system of service provision and delivery. The idea is that by such an exercise, in conjunction with an audit of existing services, duplication and inefficiency can be resolved, gaps identified and provided for, and systems set up to make services needs-led, rather than bureaucracy-dominated. A tall order! Service provision can never be a panacea. It cannot ensure that no child is ever mistreated. It is, however, an approach that really does stress the importance of prevention, so central to the work of health visitors and nurses, and is intended to avoid, wherever possible, the removal of children from their families and the harm this often does, by reducing the stresses and disadvantages that all too often lead to children being harmed or neglected.

In order to develop a co-ordinated system of service provision, the Act specifies that local authority social services departments must identify the extent to which there are children 'in need' within their area and open and maintain a register of disabled children in their area. They can seek help to do this from other agencies, including health authorities. Registration for the disabled child is not, however, a precondition for receiving help. The child, if considered 'in need', is entitled to appropriate services. Social services departments, in developing a more co-ordinated service, will need to work with others, including for example local authority housing and recreation services as well as the voluntary sector. In fulfilling this responsibility they will undoubtedly face major problems, given the constraints on their resources. At the same time, the Children Act does offer a firmer legal pressure on local authorities to take account of children's welfare in the provision and delivery of their services.

The services that can be — and in some circumstances must be — provided include day-care and after-school and holiday care, family centres, and help with laundry, holidays and housing. It also includes, as a service, the provision of accommodation. This may be foster care or, say, help to enable relatives to look after a child for a while. Its primary aim is to offer respite at times of trouble and to give families looking after children with disabilities a break. In some situations, however, it may be a long-term solution, for example to a parent's chronic mental illness. The important point about accommodating children is that it is an entirely voluntary arrangement on the part of the parent(s). If somebody with parental responsibility is willing and able to look after the child, then accommodation cannot be provided, unless the child 'in need' is over sixteen and requests it. So the parent can take the child back at any point, without consulting anybody or asking for permission. It is therefore completely different from the child being 'taken into care' — that can now only happen when a court makes an order.

Changes in the way children are protected

Of all the areas covered by the new legislation, its new provisions for child protection have received the most publicity, not least because the Bill was debated during the glare of publicity following the events in Cleveland. Prior to that, public outcry had tended to focus on the relatively small number of cases where protection had failed and children had been brutally killed — the names of Jasmine Beckford, Kimberley Carlile, Lester Chapman and Doreen Mason were much in people's minds. The events in Cleveland brought a contradictory clamour for less intervention, not more. The medical and social work professions were accused of snatching children from loving families and hiding them away until triumphantly returned by the courts. However, subsequent more rational analysis of those events, and more recent scandals like the 'pindown' inquiry and the Frank Beck case in Leicestershire, remind us that children need effective protection outside as well as within their families. What was seen to be needed was a new legislative framework which would get a better balance between providing fast and effective means to ensure the safety of children at risk of being seriously harmed, and making sure children were not needlessly and painfully separated from their families. The need to make intervention open to challenge at an early stage and to make professionals publicly accountable for the decisions they took were seen as critical. At the same time, scrutiny was seen as needing to be extended to all situations where children are cared for and live away from their families.

The Act is designed to avoid the need for enforced intervention in families to protect children. This is to be achieved in two ways: first, as we have seen, by providing services to alleviate stresses and to support families coping with difficult times and demanding children and hence prevent the need to intervene in the first place; and secondly, by trying, wherever possible, to reach voluntary agreements with parents about ways of making sure their children are safe from harm. Nonetheless, the Act also contains provisions for intervention when the need arises. Indeed, it very considerably simplifies and clarifies the legal basis under which children may be protected.

The Act places a duty on local authorities to investigate concerns about a child's safety when it is reported to them, or of which they become aware through their own casework with a family, or in circumstances where other professionals have intervened, for example the police taking a child into protection. This means that whenever somebody passes on information to social services that suggests a child may be at risk of significant harm, they are obliged to follow up those concerns. Although they have a degree of discretion, they cannot merely refuse to do anything.

In order to pursue this investigation, the Act introduces a totally new order. This is intended to tackle circumstances where there are concerns about a child, but these are long-term and to do with worries about the child's health or development rather than a matter of urgent concerns about the child's safety. This order, the *Child Assessment Order*, is designed primarily to insist that a child is examined, to find out whether or not the child is all right. For example, it might be appropriate in a case where medical staff suspect a child is developing hearing problems, yet it seems the child's parents are unwilling to take this seriously. If several clinic appointments have been missed, the health visitor is not allowed to examine the child when she visits, and the parents repeatedly refuse to bring the child to the surgery for hearing tests, then there would be grounds to believe that the child's development was being impaired by their non-co-operation. This combination of circumstances would be sufficient for an order to be sought to allow the necessary assessment to take place.

Where, however, concerns are much more urgent, a Child Assessment Order is not appropriate. For example, it should not be used to gain access to see the child whom the parents refuse to allow anybody to even see. In such a situation, if there were real worries that the child might have been injured or was being severely neglected, an *Emergency Protection Order* must be sought. The Emergency Protection Order can be used for two rather different purposes:

- by any person to deal with a crisis by removing a child immediately, or keeping the child somewhere safe (for example, a hospital ward);
- by a local authority or the NSPCC in order to allow them to conduct or continue an investigation, where there are immediate concerns about a child's safety.

The Emergency Protection Order provides the applicant, usually the local authority or NSPCC, with limited parental responsibility. However, they do not automatically have the right to authorise a medical examination or to enter premises to collect the child. To be able to do so they need, in the former case, to obtain a direction within the order specifying they may do so; and in the latter, to accompany the order with a warrant for the police to help them. If the order contains a direction that the child is to be medically examined, the child is entitled to refuse, if she or he is of sufficient understanding to make an informed decision.

Both orders, and indeed care and supervision orders too, hinge upon the concept of significant harm, which is central to the Act's approach to child protection. The Act identifies that, in every situation, the circumstances in which an order may be made are where children are, or are likely to be, 'significantly harmed'. Significant harm is defined in terms of 'harm' meaning ill-treatment, including sexual abuse and forms of ill-treatment which are not physical, or the impairment of physical or mental health or development. Development includes physical, intellectual, emotional, social or behaviourial development, and should be compared with that which would reasonably be expected of a similar child. The different orders are couched in slightly different language. In some, all that needs to be demonstrated is that the risk of significant harm is suspected; in others, that there is 'reasonable cause to believe the child is being (or likely to be) significantly harmed'. There are other subtle, but in law critical, differences. So anybody involved in seeking an order needs more detail than can be provided here and also legal advice.

The Child Assessment Order may last for up to seven days, although this may be at a specified time in the future, for example in a week's time, to allow arrangements for assessment to be set up. An Emergency Protection Order may last for eight days, with a possible extension to a further eight. However, except where parents attended the original hearing, they, or indeed the child, may challenge the order after seventy-two hours. In any case, the child must be returned as soon as it is safe to do so. Unless specified in the order, children should continue to have contact with their parents even though this may be supervised.

These orders offer, therefore, only short-term protection. Following on from them, the desired outcome is a voluntary set of arrangements, agreed with and developed in partnership with the child's parents, to make sure the child continues to be safe. If this cannot be achieved, despite genuine attempts, then other arrangements must be made. These may include applying for a care or supervision order. Under a care order, the child and parents must be consulted about where the child shall live, and this should be, as far as possible, close to home, keeping brothers and sisters together, and somewhere not unsuitable if the child has a disability. Arrangements must be made, except where specifically prohibited by the court in the order, for continued contact with parents and any others with parental responsibility.

Changes in the provision of substitute care

Fundamental to the Act is a conviction that all children deserve basic standards of care, wherever they grow up and are looked after. These include both physical and structural 'baseline' conditions and appropriate treatment and services with regard to their race, culture, religion and linguistic background. As well as making the removal of children permanently from their families a last resort only (i.e. not using it, say, as a mechanism to tackle truanting or a response to homelessness), this demands more thoughtful placement of children in care, wherever possible maintaining their links with their wider family and community. At the same time under the Act, children and their families have a greater say in deciding where and how services, including substitute care, are to be provided, and more effective recourse to complain if they are dissatisfied. Moreover, the Act includes new provisions for ensuring the safety and monitoring the standards of care for children living away from home, whether in boarding schools, hospital and nursing homes or in private foster care. Similarly, it introduces more stringent controls over the standards of day-care and better protection for children looked after in this way. The Act also acknowledges that young people who have been cared for outside their families, in children's homes, foster care, hospitals and nursing homes, are entitled to help and support in their transition into adulthood, and adequate after-care services to enable them to live independently. The Act places a duty on local authorities to befriend and support them, and in some circumstances to provide them with housing, money and other resources — for example, to help them continue their education or training.

Implications of the Act for nurses and health visitors

Clearly, the first implication is the need to be properly informed about the Act, and we hope this chapter has helped. The Act's changes in relation to 'parental responsibility' will mean that record-keeping systems must be updated, to take account of all those people (e.g. 'non-custodial parents' under previous legislation) who now have parental responsibility for children in your care. Health visitors and nurses will need to know, for each child, who has parental responsibility, and any additional information (for example, if there have been arrangements made under a Contact Order). A clear distinction needs to be made between children who are accommodated and those who are 'in care'. All of these will have implications for who, for example, may consent to medical examinations or treatment. Note too that account must be taken of the Gillick ruling, that children are able to make decisions about such things for themselves once they reach sixteen, and below that age if they are capable of making an informed decision, though advice should be sought on this.

Record-keeping will also be vital in terms of child protection. The health visitor's or nurse's carefully recorded notes, kept systematically over time, may be critical evidence about whether the child is suffering or likely to suffer 'significant harm'. Here the nurse's expertise may well be the key factor in ensuring a child is properly protected. You will need to find out more about the implications of written reports in court proceedings, and will need specific legal advice if you are directly involved. That having been said, the more child-centred court system, with the shift to local courts, should make the experience of appearing in court a lot less daunting. Courts have changed, and there has been a shift from an adversarial to a 'solution-seeking' approach. Some lawyers and magistrates, of course, have not yet fully made the change-over, but early signs indicate that, in an increasing number of courts, the Act really has signified a 'new beginning'.

At the same time, the nurse's carefully established relationship with a family may well be crucial for achieving a voluntary, negotiated set of arrangements, avoiding the need for legal intervention. Both of these indicate a need to develop and build upon links with social service staff, so that the nurse can support them in their primary responsibility for child protection.

But, more than anything else, the health visitor's and nurse's roles in preventive care will be much more significant in the new approach to child protection. In a very real sense, the Act endorses and reinforces the importance of the work undertaken by health visitors and nurses. For example, their expertise in working with children with disabilities, and helping to assess their needs for services, will be a key element in making sure those children can, as the Act directs they should, get as much out of life as other children. This kind of work may lack the 'glamour' and excitement of some of the high-profile intervention work that is sometimes needed, but the Act specifically aims to provide a framework which supports the protective ethos of this work, and values the nurse's expertise in promoting the health and wellbeing of the children and parents in the nurse's care.

The Act also, though, acknowledges that sometimes the only way to make sure a child is safe is to intervene effectively and quickly. It simplifies and clarifies what must be done in such circumstances, and provides clear and unequivocal routes to keep children safe. If you are likely ever to be involved in such a crisis, it is essential you make sure you are fully informed what you can (and cannot) do, to whom to turn for action and advice, and what support you can call upon. This will mean making sure local policies and procedures — and the essential networks of contacts — are in place and nurtured, so they can be called into play when they are needed. This means building on your links not just with social services, but with the police and your local courts. Nurse managers and child protection co-ordinators should take a lead to ensure that this happens.

At the same time, the Act does provide for the rare eventuality that, in order to protect a child, the nurse may need to act outside of the usual routes. By allowing any person to apply for an Emergency Protection Order (and this includes people like relatives or neighbours) if they can fulfil the necessary conditions, this means that the opportunity is there to act independently. In the vast majority of cases, this would be inappropriate and dysfunctional, and it makes much more sense to follow agreed and established procedures. But the Act does recognise that there may occasionally be times when this may be the only way to make sure a child is safe. In such cases you should always take legal advice if possible, but in real emergencies the local court clerk can be contacted directly.

In terms of 'children in need' once more, health (in its widest sense) and development are key concepts to establishing a child's entitlement to services, and consequently the health visitor's and nurse's work and records will play a critical role in assessment of needs. This again means building upon working relationships with social services staff, contributing both particular expertise and knowledge of the family, and services available in the local community. This may need to be done in a tactful way, since the Act places upon social services the lead role in setting up and monitoring the services and registers. Nonetheless, given the demands on their time and resources, the Act offers an opportunity for greater collaboration and co-operation — not always easy to achieve in practice, but worth while if it can lead to better services for children and their families.

Perhaps, though, the most important implication for health visitors and nurses is that the Act, despite its shortcomings, does herald a change in philosophy, making the way the law deals with children much more consistent with the nurse's own professional goals. It stresses a holistic view of the child's welfare and wellbeing, including the critical importance of a child's family, community and identity. It seeks to avoid the 'big stick' of enforced intervention, preferring to support and befriend parents when they have to cope with difficulties. It endorses and promotes a partnership style of working with families, acknowledging that even when parents may not be able to care for their children, they almost always still care about them, and, critically, children care about their parents and seldom wish to be separated totally from their family and community.

Above all, the Act seeks to treat children as people — not 'objects of professional concern' — with wishes, feelings and views of their own; and people who are entitled to respect, to a growing autonomy as they grow up, and to the services they need for a happy and healthy childhood. That has to be good news for not just children, but for all who work with them. Of course, there will be difficulties, and the frustrations of limited resources and structural and organisational problems will not be magically swept away by a change in the law. Nonetheless, the Act offers us all a chance to make things better, and that is a goal worth working for.

Index